CONTENTS

Chapter 1: Introduction to Diverticulosis — 1

Chapter 2: Anatomy and Physiology of the Gastrointestinal Tract — 21

Chapter 3: Development and Formation of Diverticula — 35

Chapter 4: Clinical Evaluation and Diagnosis — 53

Chapter 5: Complications of Diverticulosis — 69

Chapter 6: Medical Management of Diverticulosis — 92

Chapter 7: Prevention and Lifestyle Modifications — 102

Chapter 8: Holistic Approaches to Diverticulosis Management — 122

Chapter 9: Patient Education and Counseling — 143

Chapter 10: Future Directions in Diverticulosis Research — 159

CHAPTER 1: INTRODUCTION TO DIVERTICULOSIS

Definition and Overview of Diverticulosis

Diverticulosis is a common gastrointestinal condition characterized by the presence of small pouches, known as diverticula, that protrude from the wall of the colon. These diverticula typically develop in weakened areas of the colon, most commonly in the sigmoid colon, although they can occur throughout the large intestine. While diverticulosis itself may be asymptomatic, it can lead to complications such as diverticulitis, abscess formation, perforation, and obstruction, which can result in significant morbidity and mortality if left untreated.

The term "diverticulosis" is derived from the Latin words "diverticulum" (meaning "small pouch") and "-osis" (a suffix indicating a condition or state). It was first described in medical literature in the early 20th century, with the prevalence of diverticulosis increasing steadily in industrialized countries over the past century. Today, it is considered a common condition, particularly among older adults.

The exact etiology of diverticulosis remains incompletely understood, but it is believed to result from a combination of factors, including structural abnormalities in the colonic wall, increased intraluminal pressure, alterations in colonic motility, and dietary factors. The prevalence of diverticulosis tends to increase with age, with the majority of cases occurring in individuals over the age of 60. However, it can also occur in younger individuals, particularly those with predisposing risk factors such as a low-fiber diet, obesity, physical inactivity, smoking, and certain genetic predispositions.

Diverticulosis is often classified based on the severity of symptoms and the presence or absence of complications. Asymptomatic diverticulosis refers to the presence of diverticula without any associated symptoms, whereas symptomatic diverticulosis may manifest with symptoms such as abdominal pain, bloating, changes in bowel habits, and rectal bleeding. Complications of diverticulosis, such as diverticulitis, occur when the diverticula become inflamed or infected, leading to more severe symptoms and potentially life-threatening complications.

Diagnosis of diverticulosis is typically made based on a combination of clinical evaluation, imaging studies, and endoscopic procedures. Imaging modalities such as colonoscopy, computed tomography (CT) scan, and barium enema can help visualize the presence of diverticula and assess for any complications. Laboratory tests may also be performed to evaluate for signs of inflammation or infection, such as an elevated white blood cell count or C-reactive protein level.

Management of diverticulosis focuses on both symptomatic relief and prevention of complications. Dietary modifications, such as increasing fiber intake and maintaining adequate hydration, are commonly recommended to promote regular bowel movements and prevent constipation, which can exacerbate diverticular symptoms. In cases of acute diverticulitis or complications such as abscess formation or perforation, medical management with antibiotics and supportive care may be necessary, while surgical intervention may be required in severe or recurrent cases.

In summary, diverticulosis is a common gastrointestinal condition characterized by the presence of diverticula in the colon. While often asymptomatic, it can lead to complications such as diverticulitis, abscess formation, and perforation, which require prompt diagnosis and management. Understanding the definition, etiology, clinical manifestations, and management of diverticulosis is essential for healthcare providers to effectively care for patients with this condition and prevent associated complications.

Epidemiology of Diverticulosis: A Comprehensive Overview

Understanding the epidemiology of diverticulosis is essential for healthcare providers to grasp the magnitude of the condition's prevalence, its distribution across different populations, and the factors influencing its incidence. Epidemiological studies provide valuable insights into the demographic characteristics, risk factors, and trends associated with diverticulosis, enabling healthcare professionals to implement targeted prevention strategies and optimize patient care.

Prevalence and Incidence

Diverticulosis is primarily a disease of the developed world, with the prevalence varying significantly across different regions and populations. Historically, diverticulosis was more prevalent in industrialized countries such as the United States, Canada, and Western Europe. However, with changes in lifestyle and dietary habits, its prevalence has been increasing globally, including in developing nations undergoing rapid urbanization and adopting Westernized diets.

The prevalence of diverticulosis increases with age, with the majority of cases occurring in individuals over the age of 60. Studies have shown that the prevalence of diverticulosis increases with each decade of life, reaching its peak among individuals in their 80s and 90s. However, diverticulosis can also occur in younger adults, particularly those with predisposing risk factors such as obesity, physical inactivity, and a low-fiber diet.

Demographic Patterns

While diverticulosis affects both men and women, there are some differences in its demographic patterns. Historically, diverticulosis was more common in men, but recent studies suggest that the gender gap is narrowing, with similar rates observed among men and women. However, the presentation and clinical course of diverticulosis may differ between sexes, with women more likely to experience complications such as diverticulitis and bleeding.

Ethnicity may also influence the prevalence of diverticulosis, with higher rates observed among certain racial and ethnic groups. For example, diverticulosis appears to be more common among individuals of European descent compared to those of African or Asian descent. However, these differences may also reflect variations in dietary habits, lifestyle factors, and genetic predispositions among different populations.

Geographical Variations

Geographical variations in the prevalence of diverticulosis have been documented, with higher rates observed in certain regions and countries. For instance, diverticulosis is more prevalent in North America and Europe compared to Asia and Africa. Within countries, there may also be regional variations in the prevalence of diverticulosis, which may be influenced by factors such as dietary patterns, socioeconomic status, and access to healthcare.

Trends Over Time

Trends in the prevalence of diverticulosis have evolved over time, reflecting changes in population demographics, lifestyle factors, and healthcare practices. While diverticulosis was once considered a disease of the elderly, there is evidence to suggest that its incidence is increasing among younger adults. This trend has been attributed to changes in dietary habits, including decreased fiber intake and increased consumption of processed foods, as well as rising rates of obesity and sedentary lifestyles.

Risk Factors

Several risk factors have been associated with an increased risk of diverticulosis. Age is the most significant risk factor, with the prevalence of diverticulosis increasing markedly with advancing age. Other factors associated with an increased risk of diverticulosis include obesity, physical inactivity, smoking, and a low-fiber diet. Genetic predispositions may also play a role, with some studies suggesting familial clustering of diverticulosis.

Conclusion

In conclusion, diverticulosis is a common gastrointestinal condition with significant variations in its prevalence, distribution, and risk factors across different populations. While historically more prevalent in developed countries and among older adults, diverticulosis is increasingly being recognized as a global health issue affecting individuals of all ages. Understanding the epidemiology of diverticulosis is crucial for implementing preventive measures, optimizing patient care, and addressing the evolving challenges associated with this condition. Further research is needed to elucidate the underlying mechanisms driving the epidemiological trends observed and to develop effective strategies for the prevention and management of diverticulosis on a global scale.

Exploring the Multifactorial Landscape of Diverticulosis: Understanding Risk Factors

Diverticulosis is a complex gastrointestinal condition influenced by a myriad of genetic, environmental, and lifestyle factors. A thorough understanding of the risk factors associated with diverticulosis is essential for healthcare providers to identify high-risk individuals, implement targeted prevention strategies, and optimize patient care. In this comprehensive exploration, we delve into the multifactorial landscape of diverticulosis risk factors, examining their interplay and implications for disease development.

Age

Age is one of the most significant risk factors for diverticulosis, with its prevalence increasing markedly with advancing age. While diverticulosis can occur at any age, it is most commonly diagnosed in individuals over the age of 60. The aging process is associated with structural changes in the colonic wall, including collagen deposition and weakening of the muscular layer, which predispose to the formation of diverticula. Additionally, age-related alterations in colonic motility and bowel habits may contribute to the development of diverticulosis.

Dietary Factors

Dietary habits play a crucial role in the pathogenesis of diverticulosis, with low-fiber diets being strongly associated with an increased risk of disease development. Fiber deficiency leads to reduced fecal bulk and slower transit time, resulting in increased intraluminal pressure within the colon. This elevated pressure promotes the formation of diverticula in weakened areas of the colonic wall. Conversely, diets rich in fiber, fruits, vegetables, and whole grains are protective against diverticulosis by promoting regular bowel movements and preventing constipation.

Obesity

Obesity is a well-established risk factor for diverticulosis, with studies consistently demonstrating a positive association between body mass index (BMI) and the prevalence of diverticular disease. Excess adiposity, particularly visceral adipose tissue, is thought to contribute to increased intra-abdominal pressure, which can exacerbate colonic wall stress and promote the development of diverticula. Furthermore, obesity is often accompanied by dietary patterns high in processed foods and low in fiber, further exacerbating the risk of diverticulosis.

Physical Inactivity

Sedentary lifestyle and lack of physical activity have been identified as independent risk factors for diverticulosis. Regular physical activity is associated with improved colonic motility, bowel regularity, and overall gastrointestinal health. Conversely, prolonged periods of inactivity and sitting may lead to decreased bowel movement frequency, increased intra-abdominal pressure, and stagnation of stool within the colon, predisposing to diverticular formation. Incorporating regular exercise into one's daily routine is therefore essential for mitigating the risk of diverticulosis.

Smoking

Cigarette smoking has been implicated as a modifiable risk

factor for diverticulosis, with studies suggesting a dose-response relationship between smoking intensity and disease risk. Nicotine and other harmful compounds present in tobacco smoke can impair colonic blood flow, promote inflammation, and compromise the integrity of the colonic mucosa, contributing to the pathogenesis of diverticula. Smoking cessation is therefore recommended as an important preventive measure for individuals at risk of diverticulosis.

Genetic Predispositions

While environmental factors play a significant role in the development of diverticulosis, genetic predispositions also contribute to disease susceptibility. Familial clustering of diverticular disease has been observed, suggesting a hereditary component to its pathogenesis. Genome-wide association studies (GWAS) have identified several genetic variants associated with diverticulosis, including genes involved in connective tissue metabolism, inflammation, and colonic smooth muscle function. Further research is needed to elucidate the specific genetic mechanisms underlying diverticular formation and progression.

Conclusion

In conclusion, diverticulosis is a multifactorial condition influenced by a complex interplay of genetic, environmental, and lifestyle factors. Age, dietary habits, obesity, physical inactivity, smoking, and genetic predispositions all contribute to disease development through various mechanisms, including increased colonic wall stress, altered motility, and inflammation. Understanding the intricate landscape of diverticulosis risk factors is essential for implementing targeted preventive strategies and optimizing patient care. By addressing modifiable risk factors and promoting healthy lifestyle behaviors, healthcare providers can mitigate the burden of diverticular disease and improve patient outcomes.

Pathophysiology of Diverticulosis: Unraveling the Intricacies

Diverticulosis is a complex gastrointestinal disorder characterized by the presence of diverticula, small pouch-like protrusions, in the colonic wall. While traditionally thought to result from increased intraluminal pressure and structural weakness in the colonic wall, our understanding of the pathophysiology of diverticulosis has evolved to encompass a multitude of factors, including intestinal wall structure, pressure dynamics, microbiota interaction, and genetic predispositions. In this extensive exploration, we delve into each aspect of diverticulosis pathophysiology, unraveling the intricacies that contribute to its development and progression.

Intestinal Wall Structure

The structural integrity of the intestinal wall plays a pivotal role in the pathogenesis of diverticulosis. The colon consists of several layers, including the mucosa, submucosa, muscularis propria, and serosa, each contributing to its mechanical properties and function. Key components of the intestinal wall involved in diverticular formation include:

- **Mucosa**: The innermost layer of the intestinal wall, the mucosa, serves as a protective barrier against luminal contents and pathogens. Alterations in mucosal integrity, such as inflammation or injury, may predispose to diverticular formation by weakening the colonic wall and facilitating herniation of the mucosa and submucosa through the muscular layer.
- **Submucosa**: Beneath the mucosa lies the submucosa, a layer rich in blood vessels, lymphatics, and nerve

endings. Structural changes in the submucosa, such as collagen deposition or fibrosis, can impair the compliance of the colonic wall and contribute to the development of diverticula.

- **Muscularis Propria**: The muscularis propria, consisting of circular and longitudinal smooth muscle layers, is responsible for peristalsis and colonic motility. Dysfunction in smooth muscle contractility or coordination may result in increased intraluminal pressure and predispose to diverticular formation.
- **Serosa**: The outermost layer of the colon, the serosa, provides structural support and facilitates peritoneal attachment. Weakness or defects in the serosal layer may predispose to the development of true diverticula, characterized by herniation of all layers of the colonic wall.

Structural abnormalities in the colonic wall, such as focal defects in the muscularis propria or alterations in connective tissue composition, contribute to the formation of diverticula. These structural weaknesses, combined with increased intraluminal pressure, create a predisposing environment for diverticular herniation and outpouching.

Pressure Dynamics

Pressure dynamics within the colon play a central role in the pathophysiology of diverticulosis. Increased intraluminal pressure, resulting from various physiological and pathological factors, is a key contributor to diverticular formation. Several mechanisms contribute to elevated intraluminal pressure and colonic wall stress, including:

- **Decreased Colonic Compliance**: Age-related changes in colonic compliance, including decreased elasticity and increased stiffness, contribute to elevated intraluminal pressure and predispose to diverticulosis.

Reduced compliance may result from alterations in colonic smooth muscle function, changes in connective tissue composition, or alterations in neural regulation.

- **Altered Colonic Motility**: Dysregulation of colonic motility, characterized by abnormal patterns of peristalsis or impaired coordination of smooth muscle contraction, can lead to stagnation of luminal contents and increased intraluminal pressure. Conditions associated with altered colonic motility, such as irritable bowel syndrome (IBS) or neuromuscular disorders, may predispose to diverticular formation.
- **Dietary Factors**: Dietary habits, particularly low-fiber diets high in processed foods and refined carbohydrates, are associated with increased intraluminal pressure and a higher risk of diverticulosis. Fiber deficiency leads to reduced fecal bulk, slower transit time, and increased colonic fermentation, resulting in gas production and elevated intraluminal pressure.
- **Obesity**: Excess adiposity, particularly visceral adipose tissue, is associated with increased intra-abdominal pressure and mechanical stress on the colonic wall. Obesity-related factors, such as insulin resistance, adipokine dysregulation, and chronic inflammation, may further exacerbate colonic wall stress and contribute to diverticular formation.
- **Straining and Constipation**: Chronic straining during defecation, often associated with constipation or inadequate bowel habits, can lead to sustained elevations in intraluminal pressure and predispose to diverticular herniation. Straining increases the risk of colonic wall trauma and mucosal injury, further exacerbating diverticular formation.

Pressure dynamics within the colon are influenced by a complex interplay of physiological, dietary, and lifestyle factors. Elevated intraluminal pressure, coupled with structural weaknesses in the colonic wall, creates an environment conducive to diverticular formation and progression.

Microbiota Interaction

The gut microbiota, consisting of trillions of microorganisms residing in the gastrointestinal tract, plays a crucial role in the pathophysiology of diverticulosis. The microbiota interacts with the colonic mucosa, immune system, and luminal contents, influencing colonic inflammation, motility, and barrier function. Dysbiosis, characterized by alterations in the composition and function of the gut microbiota, has been implicated in the pathogenesis of diverticulosis. Key mechanisms through which the microbiota contributes to diverticular formation include:

- **Inflammation**: Dysbiosis and alterations in gut microbial composition can promote low-grade mucosal inflammation and immune activation, contributing to colonic wall damage and predisposing to diverticular formation. Inflammatory mediators released by gut bacteria, such as lipopolysaccharides (LPS) and proinflammatory cytokines, may disrupt colonic barrier function and exacerbate mucosal injury.
- **Fermentation**: The gut microbiota plays a central role in colonic fermentation, the process by which dietary fibers and complex carbohydrates are metabolized into short-chain fatty acids (SCFAs) and gases. SCFAs, particularly butyrate, serve as an energy source for colonic epithelial cells and have anti-inflammatory and mucosal protective effects. Dysbiosis and reduced microbial diversity may impair colonic fermentation

and predispose to diverticular formation.
- **Mucus Layer Integrity**: The gut microbiota interacts with the colonic mucus layer, a protective barrier that separates luminal contents from the underlying epithelium. Disruption of the mucus layer, secondary to dysbiosis or inflammation, can compromise colonic barrier function and increase susceptibility to mucosal injury and diverticular herniation.
- **Immune Activation**: Gut microbial products and metabolites can modulate immune responses within the colonic mucosa, influencing inflammation, immune cell activation, and tissue remodeling. Dysregulated immune responses, characterized by chronic low-grade inflammation or impaired mucosal healing, may contribute to diverticular formation and progression.

The gut microbiota is intricately involved in the pathophysiology of diverticulosis, with dysbiosis and microbial alterations contributing to colonic inflammation, barrier dysfunction, and mucosal injury. Targeted interventions aimed at restoring microbial homeostasis may hold promise for the prevention and management of diverticular disease.

Genetic Factors

Genetic predispositions play a significant role in the pathogenesis of diverticulosis, with familial clustering and heritability observed in affected individuals. Genome-wide association studies (GWAS) have identified several genetic variants associated with diverticular disease, implicating genes involved in connective tissue metabolism, inflammation, and colonic smooth muscle function. Key genetic factors contributing to diverticulosis include:

- **Connective Tissue Disorders**: Genetic mutations affecting connective tissue structure and integrity have been implicated in diverticular formation. Variants in genes encoding extracellular matrix proteins, such as collagen and elastin, may predispose to colonic wall weakness and herniation. Disorders associated with connective tissue abnormalities, such as Ehlers-Danlos syndrome and Marfan syndrome, are often characterized by an increased risk of diverticulosis.

- **Inflammatory Pathways**: Genetic variants in genes involved in inflammatory pathways have been associated with diverticular disease. Polymorphisms in genes encoding proinflammatory cytokines, such as tumor necrosis factor-alpha (TNF-α) and interleukin-6 (IL-6), may modulate colonic inflammation and immune responses, contributing to diverticular formation and progression. Dysregulated inflammatory signaling pathways, characterized by chronic low-grade inflammation, may promote colonic wall damage and mucosal injury.
- **Smooth Muscle Function**: Genetic mutations affecting colonic smooth muscle function and contractility have been implicated in diverticulosis. Variants in genes encoding smooth muscle proteins, such as myosin and actin, may alter colonic motility and peristalsis, predisposing to increased intraluminal pressure and diverticular herniation. Dysfunction in smooth muscle contractility may impair colonic transit and fecal evacuation, further exacerbating diverticular formation.
- **Neural Regulation**: Genetic variants affecting neural regulation of colonic motility and sensation may contribute to diverticulosis. Variants in genes encoding neurotransmitters, such as serotonin and dopamine, or their receptors, may influence colonic smooth muscle function and visceral sensitivity,

predisposing to altered bowel habits and increased intraluminal pressure. Dysregulated neural signaling pathways may disrupt colonic motility patterns and predispose to diverticular formation.

Genetic factors interact with environmental and lifestyle factors to modulate the risk of diverticulosis, highlighting the complex interplay between genetic predispositions and external influences. Further research is needed to elucidate the specific genetic mechanisms underlying diverticular formation and progression and to identify potential targets for therapeutic intervention.

Conclusion

In conclusion, the pathophysiology of diverticulosis is multifaceted, encompassing a complex interplay of intestinal wall structure, pressure dynamics, microbiota interaction, and genetic predispositions. Structural weaknesses in the colonic wall, combined with elevated intraluminal pressure and dysregulated microbial communities, create a predisposing environment for diverticular formation and herniation. Genetic factors further modulate disease susceptibility, influencing connective tissue integrity, inflammatory pathways, smooth muscle function, and neural regulation. A comprehensive understanding of diverticulosis pathophysiology is essential for guiding preventive strategies, optimizing patient care, and identifying novel therapeutic targets. Further research is needed to unravel the intricate mechanisms underlying diverticular disease and to develop targeted interventions aimed at mitigating its burden and improving patient outcomes.

Clinical Manifestations of Diverticulosis: Understanding the

Spectrum of Symptoms

Diverticulosis is a common gastrointestinal condition characterized by the presence of diverticula in the colon. While many individuals with diverticulosis remain asymptomatic, others may experience a range of clinical manifestations, varying from mild discomfort to severe complications requiring urgent medical intervention. In this comprehensive exploration, we delve into the diverse clinical manifestations of diverticulosis, shedding light on the spectrum of symptoms encountered in clinical practice.

Asymptomatic Diverticulosis

The majority of individuals with diverticulosis are asymptomatic and may remain unaware of their condition until it is incidentally discovered during diagnostic imaging or endoscopic procedures performed for unrelated reasons. Asymptomatic diverticulosis is typically benign and does not require specific treatment or intervention. However, regular monitoring and preventive measures, such as dietary modifications and lifestyle changes, may be recommended to minimize the risk of complications and improve overall gastrointestinal health.

Symptomatic Diverticulosis

Symptomatic diverticulosis refers to the presence of clinical symptoms attributable to diverticular disease, ranging from mild discomfort to more severe manifestations requiring medical attention. Common symptoms associated with symptomatic diverticulosis include:

- **Abdominal Pain**: Abdominal pain is the hallmark symptom of symptomatic diverticulosis and is typically localized to the left lower quadrant of the abdomen, corresponding to the location of the sigmoid colon where diverticula are most commonly found. The pain is often described as cramping or intermittent in nature and may be accompanied by bloating, gas, and changes in bowel habits. While the exact mechanisms underlying diverticular pain are not fully understood, hypotheses include inflammation, spasm of the colonic wall, and visceral hypersensitivity.

- **Bowel Habit Changes**: Changes in bowel habits, such as constipation, diarrhea, or alternating episodes of constipation and diarrhea, are common in individuals with symptomatic diverticulosis. These changes may be attributed to alterations in colonic motility, inflammation, and disruption of the gut microbiota. Patients may also experience urgency, tenesmus, and a sensation of incomplete evacuation, further contributing to bowel discomfort and distress.
- **Bloating and Distension**: Bloating and abdominal distension are frequently reported by individuals with symptomatic diverticulosis and may result from altered gut motility, gas accumulation, and impaired digestion. Increased intraluminal pressure within the colon, secondary to constipation or fermentation of undigested carbohydrates by colonic bacteria, may exacerbate bloating and distension symptoms. Dietary modifications, such as reducing gas-producing foods and increasing fiber intake, may help alleviate these symptoms.
- **Rectal Bleeding**: Rectal bleeding, often characterized by bright red blood in the stool or on toilet tissue, is a common complication of diverticulosis and may occur intermittently or persistently. While the majority of cases of rectal bleeding in diverticulosis are self-limited and resolve spontaneously, severe or recurrent bleeding may necessitate further evaluation

and management. The exact etiology of diverticular bleeding is multifactorial and may involve mucosal injury, erosion of blood vessels within diverticula, or inflammatory changes in the colonic mucosa.

Complications of Diverticulosis

In addition to the common symptoms associated with symptomatic diverticulosis, individuals with diverticulosis are at risk of developing complications, which may require urgent medical attention and intervention. Complications of diverticulosis include:

- **Diverticulitis**: Diverticulitis refers to inflammation or infection of one or more diverticula, typically presenting with acute onset of localized abdominal pain, fever, and leukocytosis. Complications of diverticulitis may include abscess formation, perforation, fistula formation, and bowel obstruction. Severe cases of diverticulitis may require hospitalization, intravenous antibiotics, and in some cases, surgical intervention.
- **Abscess Formation**: Abscess formation occurs when inflammatory exudate and bacteria accumulate within a diverticular pouch, leading to the formation of a localized collection of pus. Abscesses may present with fever, chills, and focal abdominal tenderness, and may require percutaneous drainage or surgical intervention for resolution.
- **Perforation and Peritonitis**: Perforation of a diverticulum can lead to leakage of colonic contents into the peritoneal cavity, resulting in peritonitis, a life-threatening condition characterized by diffuse abdominal pain, rebound tenderness, and signs of systemic inflammation. Prompt recognition and surgical intervention are essential for the management

of perforated diverticulitis and prevention of septic complications.
- **Fistula Formation**: Fistula formation may occur as a complication of diverticulitis, resulting in abnormal communications between the colon and adjacent structures, such as the bladder, vagina, or skin. Depending on the location of the fistula, patients may present with symptoms such as urinary tract infections, pneumaturia, fecaluria, or cutaneous drainage.
- **Bowel Obstruction**: Bowel obstruction may occur secondary to strictures, adhesions, or inflammatory changes associated with recurrent diverticulitis. Patients may present with symptoms of partial or complete bowel obstruction, including abdominal distension, nausea, vomiting, and obstipation. Management may involve supportive measures, such as bowel rest and decompression, or surgical intervention for definitive treatment.

Conclusion

In conclusion, diverticulosis encompasses a spectrum of clinical manifestations, ranging from asymptomatic disease to severe complications requiring urgent medical intervention. While many individuals with diverticulosis remain asymptomatic, others may experience symptoms such as abdominal pain, bowel habit changes, bloating, and rectal bleeding. Complications of diverticulosis, including diverticulitis, abscess formation, perforation, fistula formation, and bowel obstruction, can lead to significant morbidity and mortality if left untreated. Early recognition, appropriate management, and preventive measures are essential for optimizing patient outcomes and minimizing the burden of diverticular disease. Further research is needed to elucidate the underlying mechanisms contributing to the diverse clinical manifestations of diverticulosis and to develop targeted therapies aimed at improving symptom control and reducing the risk of complications.

CHAPTER 2: ANATOMY AND PHYSIOLOGY OF THE GASTROINTESTINAL TRACT

Exploring the Intricate Structure of the Colon: An In-Depth Analysis

The colon, also known as the large intestine, is a vital component of the gastrointestinal tract responsible for the absorption of water, electrolytes, and nutrients, as well as the formation and storage of feces. Its complex structure comprises multiple layers, each serving unique functions in digestion, absorption, and motility. In this comprehensive exploration, we delve into the intricate anatomy of the colon, examining its layers, blood supply, and innervation to gain a deeper understanding of its physiological roles and pathological implications.

2.1 Structure of the Colon

The colon is divided into several segments, including the cecum, ascending colon, transverse colon, descending colon, sigmoid colon, and rectum. Each segment exhibits variations in diameter, shape, and function, reflecting its distinct anatomical and physiological characteristics. The colon can be further subdivided into distinct layers, including the mucosa, submucosa, muscularis propria, and serosa, each contributing to its structural integrity and functional properties.

Layers of the Colon Wall

The colon wall is composed of four main layers, each with specialized structures and functions:

1. **Mucosa**: The innermost layer of the colon wall, the mucosa, consists of several components, including the epithelium, lamina propria, and muscularis mucosae. The epithelium is a single layer of columnar cells that line the luminal surface of the colon and is primarily responsible for absorption, secretion, and protection. The lamina propria contains blood vessels, lymphatic vessels, and immune cells, contributing to mucosal immunity and nutrient exchange. The muscularis mucosae is a thin layer of smooth muscle fibers that provides structural support and facilitates mucosal movement.
2. **Submucosa**: Beneath the mucosa lies the submucosa, a layer of connective tissue rich in blood vessels, lymphatics, and nerve fibers. The submucosa provides structural support to the mucosa and contains the submucosal plexus, part of the enteric nervous system responsible for regulating glandular secretion and blood flow.
3. **Muscularis Propria**: The muscularis propria is the thickest layer of the colon wall and consists of two layers of smooth muscle: an inner circular

layer and an outer longitudinal layer. These muscle layers coordinate rhythmic contractions, known as peristalsis, that propel fecal material through the colon toward the rectum. The muscularis propria also contains the myenteric plexus, a network of nerve fibers and ganglia that regulate colonic motility and tone.

4. **Serosa**: The outermost layer of the colon wall, the serosa, is a thin, serous membrane composed of mesothelial cells and connective tissue. The serosa provides a smooth, slippery surface that facilitates movement of the colon within the peritoneal cavity and reduces friction with surrounding structures.

The layered structure of the colon wall provides mechanical support, facilitates nutrient absorption, and regulates motility and secretion, essential for its digestive and absorptive functions.

Blood Supply and Innervation

The colon receives its blood supply from branches of the superior mesenteric artery (SMA) and the inferior mesenteric artery (IMA), which originate from the abdominal aorta. These arterial branches form an intricate network of blood vessels that supply oxygenated blood to the colon wall, mucosa, and surrounding structures. The arterial blood supply to the colon can be divided into several main arteries, including the ileocolic artery, right colic artery, middle colic artery, left colic artery, and sigmoid arteries, each supplying specific regions of the colon.

Venous drainage of the colon occurs through the corresponding veins, which ultimately drain into the portal venous system via the superior mesenteric vein and the inferior mesenteric vein. The portal venous system transports nutrient-rich blood from the gastrointestinal tract to the liver for processing and detoxification before returning it to systemic circulation.

The colon is innervated by the enteric nervous system (ENS), a complex network of neurons and ganglia embedded within the gastrointestinal wall. The ENS regulates various aspects of colonic function, including motility, secretion, and sensation, independent of central nervous system input. The ENS consists of two main plexuses: the myenteric plexus (Auerbach's plexus) located between the circular and longitudinal muscle layers of the muscularis propria, and the submucosal plexus (Meissner's plexus) situated within the submucosa. These plexuses contain sensory, motor, and interneurons that coordinate colonic motility, modulate secretion, and transmit sensory signals to the central nervous system.

In addition to the intrinsic innervation provided by the ENS, the colon receives extrinsic innervation from the autonomic nervous system, including sympathetic and parasympathetic fibers. Sympathetic innervation originates from the thoracolumbar spinal cord and modulates colonic smooth muscle tone, blood flow, and sphincter function. Parasympathetic innervation arises from the vagus nerve (cranial nerve X) and the pelvic splanchnic nerves (S2-S4) and promotes colonic motility and secretion.

The intricate network of blood vessels and nerve fibers supplying the colon ensures proper oxygenation, nutrient delivery, and regulation of gastrointestinal function. Dysfunction or disruption of the colonic blood supply or innervation may result in impaired motility, altered sensation, or ischemic injury, contributing to various gastrointestinal disorders and clinical manifestations. Understanding the vascular and neural anatomy of the colon is essential for diagnosing and managing colorectal diseases and optimizing patient outcomes.

Conclusion

In conclusion, the colon is a vital component of the gastrointestinal tract, responsible for the absorption of water, electrolytes, and nutrients, as well as the formation and storage of feces. Its complex structure comprises multiple layers, including the mucosa, submucosa, muscularis propria, and serosa, each with specialized functions in digestion, absorption, and motility. The colon receives its blood supply from branches of the superior and inferior mesenteric arteries and is innervated by the enteric nervous system and the autonomic nervous system. A thorough understanding of the anatomy and physiology of the colon is essential for diagnosing and managing colorectal diseases and optimizing patient care. Further research into the intricate mechanisms underlying colonic function and dysfunction is warranted to advance our understanding of gastrointestinal physiology and pathology.

Exploring the Multifaceted Functions of the Colon: An In-Depth Analysis

The colon, or large intestine, plays a crucial role in the digestive process, serving as the site for absorption of water, electrolytes, and nutrients, as well as the formation and storage of feces. In addition to its absorptive functions, the colon exhibits complex motility patterns essential for propelling fecal material toward the rectum and facilitating defecation. In this comprehensive exploration, we delve into the multifaceted functions of the colon, examining its roles in absorption, secretion, and motility to gain a deeper understanding of its physiological significance and clinical implications.

2.2 Function of the Colon

The colon performs several essential functions in the digestive process, including:

- Absorption of water, electrolytes, and nutrients
- Formation and storage of feces
- Regulation of bowel motility and transit
- Maintenance of colonic microbiota
- Secretion of mucus and electrolytes

Each of these functions is coordinated by intricate physiological mechanisms that ensure efficient digestion and elimination of waste products.

Absorption and Secretion

The colon is primarily responsible for the absorption of water and electrolytes from the luminal contents, as well as the secretion of mucus and electrolytes to facilitate digestion and maintain colonic integrity.

- **Water Absorption**: The colon absorbs water from the luminal contents through osmosis, driven by the concentration gradient between the luminal fluid and the vascular compartment. The absorption of water is facilitated by specialized transporters, such as aquaporins, located on the apical and basolateral membranes of colonic epithelial cells. Water absorption is essential for maintaining hydration status and electrolyte balance, as well as forming solid feces for excretion.
- **Electrolyte Absorption**: In addition to water, the colon absorbs electrolytes, including sodium, chloride, and potassium, from the luminal contents. Electrolyte absorption occurs via passive diffusion and active transport mechanisms mediated by ion channels and transporters expressed on the surface of colonic

epithelial cells. The absorption of electrolytes is tightly regulated to maintain fluid and electrolyte homeostasis and prevent dehydration and electrolyte imbalances.

- **Nutrient Absorption**: While the small intestine is the primary site for nutrient absorption, the colon also plays a role in the absorption of certain nutrients, such as short-chain fatty acids (SCFAs) produced by colonic fermentation of dietary fibers. SCFAs, including acetate, propionate, and butyrate, serve as energy sources for colonic epithelial cells and have various metabolic and immunomodulatory effects. The absorption of SCFAs is facilitated by specific transporters expressed on colonic epithelial cells.
- **Mucus Secretion**: The colon secretes mucus, a viscous gel-like substance composed of mucins, glycoproteins, and water, which forms a protective barrier over the colonic mucosa. Mucus secretion is regulated by goblet cells, specialized epithelial cells scattered throughout the colonic mucosa, which produce and release mucus in response to luminal stimuli and microbial interactions. Mucus serves several functions, including lubricating the colonic epithelium, protecting against mechanical and chemical damage, and providing a substrate for microbial colonization.
- **Electrolyte Secretion**: In addition to mucus, the colon secretes electrolytes, such as bicarbonate and chloride ions, to maintain colonic pH and osmolarity. Electrolyte secretion is regulated by ion transporters and channels expressed on the surface of colonic epithelial cells, which modulate ion flux across the epithelial barrier. Electrolyte secretion may be stimulated by various factors, including luminal pH, osmolarity, and microbial metabolites.

The coordinated balance of absorption and secretion in the colon is essential for maintaining fluid and electrolyte homeostasis, protecting the colonic mucosa, and facilitating efficient digestion and elimination of waste products.

Motility

Colonic motility refers to the rhythmic contractions of the colonic smooth muscle, which propel fecal material through the colon toward the rectum and facilitate defecation. Motility patterns in the colon are regulated by a complex interplay of neural, hormonal, and mechanical factors, which coordinate peristaltic contractions, segmental contractions, and relaxation of the internal and external anal sphincters.

- **Peristalsis**: Peristalsis is a coordinated wave-like movement of the colonic smooth muscle that propels fecal material distally through the colon. Peristaltic contractions are initiated by the enteric nervous system (ENS), a complex network of neurons and ganglia embedded within the colonic wall, which coordinates smooth muscle contraction and relaxation. Peristalsis is regulated by neurotransmitters, such as acetylcholine and serotonin, which act on smooth muscle cells to stimulate contraction and promote colonic transit.
- **Segmental Contractions**: Segmental contractions are localized contractions of the colonic smooth muscle that mix and churn luminal contents, facilitating absorption of water and nutrients and promoting homogenization of fecal material. Segmental contractions are regulated by neural and hormonal signals, as well as intrinsic pacemaker cells known as interstitial cells of Cajal (ICC), which generate rhythmic electrical activity in the colonic wall.
- **Defecation Reflex**: Defecation is a complex

physiological process that involves the coordinated relaxation of the internal anal sphincter, contraction of the rectal smooth muscle, and voluntary control of the external anal sphincter. The defecation reflex is initiated by distention of the rectum, which activates sensory receptors in the rectal wall and triggers afferent signals to the sacral spinal cord. Efferent signals are then transmitted back to the colon and rectum via parasympathetic nerves, stimulating contraction of the rectal smooth muscle and relaxation of the internal anal sphincter.

- **Voluntary Control**: While the defecation reflex is primarily mediated by autonomic and enteric nervous system pathways, voluntary control of defecation is also important for regulating the timing and frequency of bowel movements. Voluntary control is mediated by higher centers in the brain, including the cerebral cortex and brainstem, which receive input from sensory receptors in the rectum and transmit signals to the external anal sphincter to initiate or inhibit defecation.

Colonic motility is influenced by various factors, including dietary habits, physical activity, hormonal signals, and neural modulation, which collectively regulate colonic transit, fecal propulsion, and defecation. Dysfunction or dysregulation of colonic motility can lead to gastrointestinal disorders, such as constipation, diarrhea, and irritable bowel syndrome (IBS), which can significantly impact patient quality of life and overall gastrointestinal health.

Conclusion

In conclusion, the colon performs several essential functions in the digestive process, including absorption of water, electrolytes, and nutrients, as well as the formation and storage of feces. Its complex anatomy and physiology enable efficient digestion and elimination of waste products, regulated by intricate mechanisms of absorption, secretion, and motility. Understanding the multifaceted functions of the colon is essential for diagnosing and managing gastrointestinal disorders and optimizing patient care. Further research into the underlying mechanisms of colonic function and dysfunction is warranted to advance our understanding of gastrointestinal physiology and pathology.

Exploring the Dynamic Interaction Between the Colon and its Microbiota: A Comprehensive Analysis

The colon, or large intestine, harbors a diverse and dynamic community of microorganisms collectively known as the gut microbiota. This complex ecosystem plays a fundamental role in maintaining colonic homeostasis, modulating host immune responses, and influencing various aspects of human health and disease. In this comprehensive exploration, we delve into the intricate interaction between the colon and its microbiota, examining the mechanisms of microbial colonization, host-microbe crosstalk, and the impact of dysbiosis on colonic function and health.

Microbiota Interaction

The gut microbiota comprises trillions of microorganisms, including bacteria, archaea, fungi, and viruses, which inhabit the gastrointestinal tract, with the colon hosting the highest microbial density and diversity. The composition and diversity of the colonic microbiota are influenced by various factors, including host genetics, diet, lifestyle, and environmental exposures. The dynamic interaction between the colon and its microbiota is characterized by mutualistic symbiosis, wherein host-derived nutrients support microbial growth and metabolism, while microbial-derived products modulate host physiology and immune function.

Microbial Colonization of the Colon

Microbial colonization of the colon begins shortly after birth and is influenced by maternal factors, such as mode of delivery, breastfeeding, and maternal diet. The initial microbial colonization of the neonatal gut is characterized by low diversity and abundance of microbial species, dominated by facultative anaerobes such as Enterobacteriaceae and Streptococcaceae. Over time, the colonic microbiota undergoes dynamic changes in response to dietary transitions, microbial competition, and host immune development, leading to the establishment of a stable and resilient microbial community.

The colonic microbiota is primarily composed of anaerobic bacteria, including members of the Firmicutes, Bacteroidetes, Actinobacteria, and Proteobacteria phyla, which play key roles in nutrient metabolism, immune regulation, and mucosal homeostasis. Bacterial taxa such as Bacteroides, Prevotella, Faecalibacterium, and Ruminococcus are commonly found in the colonic microbiota and contribute to its functional diversity and metabolic versatility.

Host-Microbe Crosstalk

The interaction between the colon and its microbiota is bidirectional, with host-derived signals influencing microbial composition and activity, and microbial-derived products modulating host physiology and immune function. Several mechanisms mediate host-microbe crosstalk in the colon, including:

- **Nutrient Utilization**: The colonic microbiota

metabolizes complex dietary carbohydrates, fibers, and proteins that are indigestible by the host, producing short-chain fatty acids (SCFAs), such as acetate, propionate, and butyrate, as metabolic byproducts. SCFAs serve as energy sources for colonic epithelial cells, regulate immune responses, and modulate intestinal barrier function, contributing to colonic health and homeostasis.

- **Mucosal Barrier Integrity**: The colonic microbiota interacts with the colonic mucosa, forming a dynamic interface known as the mucosal microbiota. Microbial-derived metabolites, such as SCFAs, regulate mucin production, tight junction integrity, and antimicrobial peptide expression, maintaining mucosal barrier function and protecting against pathogen invasion and inflammation.
- **Immune Regulation**: The colonic microbiota modulates host immune responses through interactions with mucosal immune cells, including dendritic cells, macrophages, and T cells. Commensal bacteria promote the development of regulatory T cells (Tregs) and anti-inflammatory cytokines, such as interleukin-10 (IL-10) and transforming growth factor-beta (TGF-β), which suppress excessive immune activation and maintain immune tolerance to luminal antigens.
- **Metabolic Regulation**: The colonic microbiota influences host metabolism through the production of microbial-derived metabolites, such as SCFAs, bile acids, and amino acids, which regulate energy metabolism, lipid homeostasis, and glucose metabolism. Dysbiosis, characterized by alterations in microbial composition and function, has been implicated in metabolic disorders, such as obesity, insulin resistance, and non-alcoholic fatty liver disease

(NAFLD).
- **Neuroendocrine Signaling**: The colonic microbiota communicates with the host nervous system through the gut-brain axis, a bidirectional communication network linking the gut microbiota, enteric nervous system (ENS), and central nervous system (CNS). Microbial-derived metabolites, such as SCFAs and neurotransmitters, modulate neuronal signaling, neurotransmitter synthesis, and brain function, influencing mood, behavior, and cognition.
- **Gut-Brain Axis**: The gut microbiota influences brain function and behavior through the gut-brain axis, a bidirectional communication network linking the gut microbiota, enteric nervous system (ENS), and central nervous system (CNS). Microbial-derived metabolites, such as SCFAs and neurotransmitters, modulate neuronal signaling, neurotransmitter synthesis, and brain function, influencing mood, behavior, and cognition.

Impact of Dysbiosis on Colonic Function and Health

Dysbiosis, characterized by alterations in microbial composition, diversity, and function, has been implicated in the pathogenesis of various gastrointestinal disorders, including inflammatory bowel disease (IBD), irritable bowel syndrome (IBS), colorectal cancer, and infectious colitis. Dysbiosis can disrupt colonic homeostasis, impair mucosal barrier function, dysregulate immune responses, and promote inflammation, contributing to disease progression and symptom severity.

Several factors can contribute to dysbiosis in the colon, including antibiotic use, dietary changes, lifestyle factors, chronic stress, and underlying medical conditions. Strategies aimed at restoring microbial balance and promoting a healthy colonic microbiota, such as dietary modifications, prebiotics, probiotics, and fecal microbiota transplantation (FMT), hold promise for the prevention and management of gastrointestinal disorders associated with dysbiosis.

Conclusion

In conclusion, the interaction between the colon and its microbiota is a dynamic and multifaceted process that plays a fundamental role in maintaining colonic homeostasis and influencing host physiology and health. The colon harbors a diverse and dynamic microbial community that modulates host immune responses, regulates mucosal barrier function, and influences various aspects of host metabolism and neuroendocrine signaling. Dysbiosis, characterized by alterations in microbial composition and function, has been implicated in the pathogenesis of gastrointestinal disorders and other systemic diseases. Understanding the intricate interplay between the colon and its microbiota is essential for elucidating the mechanisms of disease pathogenesis and developing targeted interventions aimed at restoring microbial balance and promoting colonic health. Further research into the complex interactions between host and microbial factors in the colon is warranted to advance our understanding of gastrointestinal physiology and pathology.

CHAPTER 3: DEVELOPMENT AND FORMATION OF DIVERTICULA

Unraveling the Mechanisms Behind Diverticula Formation: A Comprehensive Examination

Diverticulosis, a common gastrointestinal condition characterized by the presence of diverticula in the colon, is believed to arise from a complex interplay of structural, mechanical, and dietary factors. Understanding the mechanisms underlying diverticula formation is crucial for elucidating its pathophysiology and guiding preventive and therapeutic strategies. In this comprehensive exploration, we delve into the intricate mechanisms of diverticula formation, examining the roles of colonic wall weakness, increased intraluminal pressure, and dietary factors in the development of diverticular disease.

3.1 Mechanisms of Diverticula Formation

Diverticula, small pouch-like protrusions that develop along the colonic wall, are thought to arise from a combination of structural abnormalities, alterations in colonic motility, and dietary habits. The mechanisms underlying diverticula formation are multifactorial and involve a complex interplay of intrinsic and extrinsic factors that predispose to colonic herniation and outpouching.

Colonic Wall Weakness

Colonic wall weakness is considered a central factor in the pathogenesis of diverticula formation. The colon is composed of multiple layers, including the mucosa, submucosa, muscularis propria, and serosa, each contributing to its structural integrity and mechanical properties. Weakness in the colonic wall may result from defects in the connective tissue, smooth muscle dysfunction, or alterations in extracellular matrix components.

- **Connective Tissue Abnormalities**: Genetic predispositions and acquired connective tissue disorders, such as Ehlers-Danlos syndrome and Marfan syndrome, are associated with an increased risk of diverticulosis. Mutations in genes encoding extracellular matrix proteins, such as collagen and elastin, may impair colonic wall strength and elasticity, predisposing to herniation and outpouching.
- **Smooth Muscle Dysfunction**: Dysfunction in colonic smooth muscle contractility and motility may contribute to diverticula formation. Alterations in neural regulation, smooth muscle tone, and peristaltic activity may lead to dysmotility disorders, such as colonic inertia and hypomotility, which increase intraluminal pressure and promote herniation of the colonic wall.
- **Extracellular Matrix Remodeling**: Imbalance in

extracellular matrix remodeling processes, such as collagen deposition and degradation, may disrupt colonic wall integrity and predispose to diverticula formation. Chronic inflammation, oxidative stress, and age-related changes in tissue homeostasis may contribute to extracellular matrix alterations and weaken the colonic wall.

Increased Intraluminal Pressure

Increased intraluminal pressure within the colon is a key mechanical factor driving diverticula formation. Elevated intraluminal pressure may result from alterations in colonic motility, dietary habits, and fecal characteristics, leading to focal areas of high pressure and herniation of the colonic wall.

- **Colonic Motility Disorders**: Dysregulated colonic motility patterns, such as prolonged colonic transit time, ineffective peristalsis, and segmental contractions, may predispose to the development of diverticula. Abnormalities in neural regulation, smooth muscle function, and enteric neurotransmitter signaling may disrupt colonic motility and promote focal areas of increased pressure.
- **Constipation and Fecal Impaction**: Chronic constipation, characterized by infrequent bowel movements and difficult passage of stool, is a common risk factor for diverticulosis. Fecal impaction, resulting from retained fecal material in the colon, increases intraluminal pressure and promotes herniation of the colonic wall. Straining during defecation further exacerbates intraluminal pressure and predisposes to diverticular formation.
- **High-Fiber Diet**: Dietary habits play a crucial role in the pathogenesis of diverticulosis, with low-fiber diets associated with an increased risk of diverticular

disease. Fiber deficiency leads to the production of small, hard stools that require increased colonic pressure for propulsion, promoting herniation of the colonic wall. Conversely, high-fiber diets promote soft, bulky stools and facilitate regular bowel movements, reducing the risk of diverticula formation.

Dietary Factors

Dietary factors play a central role in the development and progression of diverticulosis. The composition, consistency, and frequency of dietary intake influence colonic motility, fecal characteristics, and intraluminal pressure, which in turn impact the risk of diverticular disease.

- **Fiber Intake**: Dietary fiber, primarily derived from fruits, vegetables, whole grains, and legumes, plays a crucial role in maintaining colonic health and preventing diverticula formation. Insufficient fiber intake results in the production of small, hard stools that require increased colonic pressure for propulsion, promoting herniation of the colonic wall. Adequate fiber intake promotes soft, bulky stools and facilitates regular bowel movements, reducing the risk of diverticulosis.
- **Fluid Intake**: Adequate fluid intake is essential for maintaining hydration and promoting soft, bulky stools, which facilitate regular bowel movements and reduce the risk of diverticula formation. Dehydration and inadequate fluid intake can lead to the production of dry, hard stools that increase intraluminal pressure and promote colonic herniation.
- **Red Meat and Processed Foods**: Consumption of red meat and processed foods, which are low in fiber and high in fat and refined carbohydrates, has been associated with an increased risk of

diverticular disease. These dietary patterns promote the production of small, hard stools and alter colonic microbiota composition, which may predispose to diverticula formation and exacerbate symptoms of diverticulosis.
- **Alcohol and Caffeine**: Excessive alcohol consumption and caffeine intake have been implicated in the pathogenesis of diverticulosis. Alcohol and caffeine act as diuretics, promoting dehydration and increasing colonic transit time, which may lead to alterations in fecal consistency and intraluminal pressure. Moderation of alcohol and caffeine consumption is recommended to reduce the risk of diverticular disease.

Conclusion

In conclusion, diverticula formation in the colon is a multifactorial process involving a complex interplay of structural, mechanical, and dietary factors. Weakness in the colonic wall, increased intraluminal pressure, and dietary habits contribute to the development and progression of diverticulosis. Understanding the mechanisms underlying diverticula formation is essential for guiding preventive and therapeutic strategies aimed at reducing the burden of diverticular disease and improving patient outcomes. Further research into the pathophysiology of diverticulosis and the role of dietary interventions in disease prevention is warranted to advance our understanding of this common gastrointestinal condition.

The Role of Aging in Diverticular Disease: A Critical Examination

As individuals age, they become increasingly susceptible to various health conditions, including gastrointestinal disorders such as diverticular disease. Understanding the role of aging in the pathogenesis, progression, and management of diverticulosis is essential for optimizing clinical care and improving patient outcomes. In this discourse, we explore the multifaceted impact of aging on diverticular disease, examining the physiological changes, risk factors, and clinical implications associated with aging in the context of diverticulosis.

Physiological Changes Associated with Aging

Aging is characterized by a myriad of physiological changes that affect multiple organ systems, including the gastrointestinal tract. In the colon, advancing age is associated with alterations in colonic motility, changes in mucosal integrity, and increased susceptibility to inflammation and injury. These age-related changes can predispose individuals to the development of diverticula and exacerbate symptoms of diverticular disease.

- **Colonic Motility**: Aging is associated with changes in colonic motility patterns, including decreased smooth muscle contractility, impaired peristalsis, and delayed colonic transit time. These alterations in colonic motility can lead to constipation, fecal stasis, and increased intraluminal pressure, which are key risk factors for diverticula formation.
- **Mucosal Integrity**: Aging is also associated with alterations in colonic mucosal integrity, including thinning of the mucosal layer, decreased mucin production, and impaired barrier function. These changes can compromise the protective barrier of the colonic mucosa, increasing susceptibility to inflammation, injury, and diverticular disease.
- **Immune Function**: Aging is characterized by changes in immune function, including immunosenescence

and chronic low-grade inflammation, often referred to as inflammaging. Age-related alterations in immune function can impair mucosal immunity, increase susceptibility to infections, and exacerbate inflammatory responses in the colon, contributing to the pathogenesis of diverticular disease.

Risk Factors for Diverticular Disease in the Elderly

Several factors contribute to the increased risk of diverticular disease in the elderly population, including age-related changes in colonic physiology, dietary habits, comorbidities, and medication use. Understanding these risk factors is crucial for identifying high-risk individuals and implementing targeted preventive strategies.

- **Decreased Colonic Motility**: Age-related changes in colonic motility, including decreased smooth muscle contractility and impaired peristalsis, increase the risk of fecal stasis and diverticula formation. Constipation, a common symptom of aging, is associated with increased intraluminal pressure and predisposes individuals to diverticular disease.
- **Dietary Habits**: Dietary habits play a significant role in the development and progression of diverticular disease, particularly in the elderly population. Low-fiber diets, common among older adults, are associated with increased risk of diverticulosis and diverticulitis. Insufficient fiber intake leads to the production of small, hard stools that require increased colonic pressure for propulsion, promoting herniation of the colonic wall and diverticular formation.
- **Comorbidities**: Elderly individuals often have multiple comorbidities, such as cardiovascular disease, diabetes, and chronic kidney disease, which can predispose to diverticular disease. These comorbid

conditions may impact colonic physiology, immune function, and medication use, increasing the risk of diverticular complications and adverse outcomes.

- **Medication Use**: Elderly individuals are more likely to use medications that affect colonic motility, including opioids, anticholinergic agents, and calcium channel blockers. These medications can impair colonic transit, promote constipation, and increase the risk of diverticular disease. Polypharmacy, common among older adults, further exacerbates the risk of medication-related adverse effects on colonic function.

Clinical Implications of Aging in Diverticular Disease

Aging poses several clinical challenges in the management of diverticular disease, including diagnostic considerations, treatment strategies, and preventive interventions. Older adults may present with atypical symptoms, comorbid conditions, and age-related changes in colonic physiology that influence disease presentation and management.

- **Diagnostic Challenges**: Older adults with diverticular disease may present with atypical symptoms, such as altered bowel habits, abdominal discomfort, and nonspecific symptoms of frailty. Diagnostic evaluation in the elderly population requires a comprehensive approach, including clinical assessment, imaging studies, and consideration of age-related comorbidities.
- **Treatment Strategies**: Treatment of diverticular disease in the elderly population should be tailored to individual patient characteristics, including age, comorbidities, and functional status. Conservative management, including dietary modifications, fiber supplementation, and symptom management, is often recommended as first-line therapy. In cases

of complicated diverticulitis or recurrent symptoms, surgical intervention may be indicated, taking into account the patient's overall health and life expectancy.
- **Preventive Interventions**: Preventive interventions aimed at reducing the risk of diverticular disease in older adults focus on promoting healthy lifestyle habits, including adequate fiber intake, hydration, and physical activity. Screening for age-related comorbidities, such as cardiovascular disease and diabetes, may also help identify individuals at higher risk of diverticular complications and guide preventive strategies.

Conclusion

In conclusion, aging plays a significant role in the pathogenesis, progression, and management of diverticular disease. Age-related changes in colonic physiology, dietary habits, comorbidities, and medication use contribute to the increased risk of diverticula formation and complications in older adults. Understanding the physiological changes associated with aging and their impact on diverticular disease is essential for optimizing clinical care and improving outcomes in elderly patients. Further research into the mechanisms of diverticular disease in the elderly population is warranted to develop targeted interventions aimed at reducing the burden of this common gastrointestinal condition.

Deciphering the Genetic Landscape of Diverticular Disease: Insights and Implications

The role of genetics in the pathogenesis of diverticular disease has garnered increasing attention in recent years, shedding light on the complex interplay between genetic susceptibility, environmental factors, and colonic physiology. Understanding the genetic underpinnings of diverticular disease is crucial for unraveling its etiology, identifying high-risk individuals, and developing targeted preventive and therapeutic strategies. In this exploration, we delve into the multifaceted role of genetics in diverticular disease, examining genetic risk factors, heritability estimates, and potential implications for clinical practice.

Genetic Risk Factors for Diverticular Disease

Genetic studies have identified several genetic variants and susceptibility loci associated with diverticular disease, providing valuable insights into its underlying pathophysiology and etiology. These genetic risk factors encompass a wide range of biological pathways, including connective tissue integrity, colonic motility, inflammation, and immune regulation.

- **Connective Tissue Genes**: Variants in genes encoding extracellular matrix proteins, such as collagen and elastin, have been implicated in the pathogenesis of diverticular disease. Mutations in collagen genes COL1A1 and COL3A1, which play key roles in colonic wall integrity and elasticity, have been associated with an increased risk of diverticulosis and diverticulitis. These genetic variants may predispose individuals to colonic wall weakness and herniation, leading to diverticula formation.
- **Colonic Motility Genes**: Genetic variants affecting colonic smooth muscle function and motility have also been implicated in diverticular disease. Polymorphisms in genes encoding neurotransmitter receptors, ion channels, and signaling molecules involved in enteric nervous system (ENS) function,

such as serotonin receptor 5-HT4 and potassium channel KCNN3, have been associated with altered colonic motility and increased risk of diverticulosis.

- **Inflammatory Genes**: Inflammation plays a crucial role in the pathogenesis of diverticular disease, with genetic variants in inflammatory genes contributing to disease susceptibility. Variants in genes encoding pro-inflammatory cytokines, such as tumor necrosis factor-alpha (TNF-α) and interleukin-6 (IL-6), have been implicated in the development and progression of diverticulitis. These genetic variants may modulate immune responses, mucosal inflammation, and susceptibility to diverticular complications.
- **Immune Regulation Genes**: Dysregulated immune responses and impaired mucosal immunity have been implicated in the pathogenesis of diverticular disease, with genetic variants in immune regulation genes contributing to disease susceptibility. Variants in genes encoding toll-like receptors (TLRs), nucleotide-binding oligomerization domain (NOD)-like receptors, and regulatory T cells (Tregs) have been associated with altered immune function and increased risk of diverticulitis.

Heritability Estimates and Familial Aggregation

Family-based studies and twin studies have provided valuable insights into the heritability of diverticular disease and the degree of familial aggregation observed in affected individuals. Heritability estimates suggest that genetic factors contribute to approximately 40-50% of the overall risk of diverticular disease, with environmental factors accounting for the remaining variance.

- **Family History**: Individuals with a family history of diverticular disease have an increased risk of developing the condition themselves, suggesting a genetic predisposition to disease susceptibility. First-degree relatives of individuals with diverticular disease are at higher risk of developing diverticulosis and diverticulitis, indicating familial aggregation of the disease phenotype.

- **Twin Studies**: Twin studies have provided further evidence of the genetic contribution to diverticular disease, with monozygotic twins demonstrating a higher concordance rate for disease phenotype compared to dizygotic twins. These findings support the role of genetic factors in disease susceptibility and highlight the importance of genetic predisposition in the pathogenesis of diverticular disease.

Clinical Implications and Future Directions

The identification of genetic risk factors for diverticular disease has important implications for clinical practice, including risk stratification, screening, and personalized management strategies. Genetic testing and risk assessment may help identify individuals at higher risk of developing diverticular disease and guide preventive interventions aimed at reducing disease burden and complications.

- **Risk Stratification**: Genetic risk stratification may help identify individuals at higher risk of developing diverticular disease and guide targeted preventive strategies, such as lifestyle modifications, dietary interventions, and pharmacological interventions aimed at reducing disease risk and severity.
- **Screening Programs**: Genetic screening programs targeting high-risk individuals may facilitate early detection and intervention for diverticular disease, potentially reducing the incidence of diverticular complications and improving patient outcomes.

- **Personalized Management**: Personalized management strategies based on individual genetic profiles may help optimize clinical care and improve treatment outcomes for patients with diverticular disease. Tailored interventions, such as dietary counseling, pharmacogenomics-guided therapy, and genetic counseling, may enhance patient adherence and response to treatment.

Conclusion

In conclusion, genetics plays a significant role in the pathogenesis of diverticular disease, with genetic variants and susceptibility loci contributing to disease susceptibility and phenotype. Understanding the genetic underpinnings of diverticular disease is crucial for elucidating its etiology, identifying high-risk individuals, and developing targeted preventive and therapeutic strategies. Further research into the genetic determinants of diverticular disease and their impact on disease pathogenesis and management is warranted to advance our understanding of this common gastrointestinal condition and improve patient care.

Microbiota Dysbiosis in Diverticular Disease: Unraveling the Complex Interplay

The gut microbiota, comprising trillions of microorganisms, plays a pivotal role in maintaining colonic homeostasis and modulating host physiology. Dysbiosis, characterized by alterations in microbial composition, diversity, and function, has been implicated in the pathogenesis and progression of various gastrointestinal disorders, including diverticular disease. In this exploration, we delve into the intricate relationship between microbiota dysbiosis and diverticular disease, examining the mechanisms, clinical implications, and therapeutic interventions associated with microbial imbalance in the colon.

Microbial Dysbiosis in Diverticular Disease

Emerging evidence suggests that diverticular disease is associated with alterations in colonic microbial composition and function, leading to microbial dysbiosis and disruption of host-microbe interactions. Dysbiosis in diverticular disease is characterized by shifts in microbial diversity, depletion of beneficial commensal bacteria, and expansion of pathogenic microorganisms, contributing to inflammation, mucosal injury, and disease progression.

- **Decreased Microbial Diversity**: Patients with diverticular disease often exhibit reduced microbial diversity in the colon, characterized by a decrease in the abundance and richness of microbial taxa. This loss of microbial diversity is associated with alterations in colonic physiology, impaired mucosal barrier function, and increased susceptibility to inflammation and infection.
- **Alterations in Microbial Composition**: Dysbiosis in diverticular disease is marked by alterations in the relative abundance of specific microbial taxa, including Firmicutes, Bacteroidetes, and Proteobacteria. Changes in microbial composition, such as increased abundance of pathogenic bacteria and depletion of beneficial commensals, may contribute to colonic inflammation, mucosal injury, and disease exacerbation.
- **Disruption of Host-Microbe Interactions**: Dysbiosis disrupts the delicate balance between the colonic microbiota and the host immune system, leading to

dysregulated immune responses, impaired mucosal immunity, and chronic inflammation. Altered host-microbe interactions in diverticular disease may promote the development of diverticulitis, exacerbate symptoms, and increase the risk of complications.

Mechanisms of Microbiota Dysbiosis in Diverticular Disease

Several factors contribute to microbiota dysbiosis in diverticular disease, including dietary habits, colonic motility disorders, mucosal inflammation, and antibiotic use. Understanding these mechanisms is essential for elucidating the pathogenesis of dysbiosis and identifying potential targets for therapeutic intervention.

- **Dietary Habits**: Dietary factors play a crucial role in shaping the composition and function of the colonic microbiota, with high-fat, low-fiber diets associated with increased risk of dysbiosis and diverticular disease. Insufficient fiber intake leads to microbial imbalance, reduced microbial diversity, and expansion of pathogenic bacteria, predisposing to inflammation and mucosal injury.
- **Colonic Motility Disorders**: Dysregulated colonic motility patterns, such as constipation and fecal stasis, promote dysbiosis by altering colonic transit time, fecal composition, and microbial metabolism. Prolonged colonic transit time and fecal retention create an anaerobic environment conducive to the growth of pathogenic bacteria and the depletion of beneficial commensals, exacerbating microbial imbalance and inflammation.
- **Mucosal Inflammation**: Chronic inflammation in the colon, a hallmark of diverticular disease, disrupts mucosal integrity, impairs immune function, and alters microbial composition. Inflammatory

mediators, such as interleukin-6 (IL-6) and tumor necrosis factor-alpha (TNF-α), promote dysbiosis by modulating microbial growth, adherence, and virulence, leading to microbial imbalance and disease exacerbation.
- **Antibiotic Use**: Antibiotic therapy, commonly prescribed for diverticulitis and diverticular bleeding, disrupts the colonic microbiota and promotes dysbiosis by eliminating beneficial commensal bacteria, altering microbial diversity, and facilitating the overgrowth of pathogenic microorganisms. Prolonged or repeated antibiotic exposure may exacerbate dysbiosis, impair mucosal healing, and increase the risk of recurrent diverticular disease.

Clinical Implications and Therapeutic Interventions

The recognition of microbiota dysbiosis as a key pathogenic factor in diverticular disease has important implications for clinical practice, including diagnostic strategies, treatment modalities, and preventive interventions aimed at restoring microbial balance and promoting colonic health.

- **Microbiota Analysis**: Microbiota analysis, including microbial profiling and functional characterization, may help identify microbial signatures associated with diverticular disease and guide personalized treatment strategies. High-throughput sequencing techniques, such as 16S rRNA gene sequencing and metagenomic sequencing, enable comprehensive assessment of microbial composition and function in the colon.
- **Probiotics and Prebiotics**: Probiotics and prebiotics, dietary supplements containing beneficial bacteria or substrates that selectively stimulate their growth, have been proposed as therapeutic interventions for diverticular disease. Probiotics, such as Lactobacillus

and Bifidobacterium species, may restore microbial balance, modulate immune responses, and reduce inflammation in the colon. Prebiotics, such as soluble fibers and oligosaccharides, promote the growth of beneficial commensals, enhance mucosal barrier function, and alleviate symptoms of diverticular disease.

- **Fecal Microbiota Transplantation (FMT)**: Fecal microbiota transplantation (FMT), the transfer of fecal microbiota from a healthy donor to a recipient, has emerged as a potential therapeutic option for recurrent or refractory diverticular disease. FMT aims to restore microbial balance, replenish beneficial commensals, and promote colonic healing by modulating host-microbe interactions and immune responses.
- **Dietary Modification**: Dietary modification, including increased fiber intake, reduced fat consumption, and avoidance of dietary triggers, plays a crucial role in the management of diverticular disease and microbiota dysbiosis. High-fiber diets promote microbial diversity, enhance colonic motility, and reduce inflammation, whereas low-fiber diets exacerbate dysbiosis, impair mucosal healing, and increase the risk of diverticular complications.

Conclusion

In conclusion, microbiota dysbiosis plays a significant role in the pathogenesis and progression of diverticular disease, contributing to inflammation, mucosal injury, and disease exacerbation. Understanding the mechanisms underlying dysbiosis and its clinical implications is essential for developing targeted therapeutic interventions aimed at restoring microbial balance and promoting colonic health in patients with diverticular disease. Further research into the role of microbiota dysbiosis in diverticular disease pathogenesis and treatment is warranted to advance our understanding of this common gastrointestinal condition and improve patient outcomes.

CHAPTER 4: CLINICAL EVALUATION AND DIAGNOSIS

Deciphering the Signs and Symptoms of Diverticular Disease: A Comprehensive Analysis

Diverticular disease, encompassing diverticulosis and diverticulitis, presents with a spectrum of signs and symptoms ranging from asymptomatic diverticulosis to potentially life-threatening diverticulitis complications. Understanding the clinical manifestations of diverticular disease is crucial for accurate diagnosis, risk stratification, and appropriate management. In this comprehensive analysis, we explore the diverse array of signs and symptoms associated with diverticular disease, examining their pathophysiology, diagnostic relevance, and clinical implications.

4.1 Signs and Symptoms

Diverticular disease encompasses a wide range of signs and symptoms, which vary in severity and presentation depending on the underlying pathology, disease stage, and individual patient factors. Common manifestations include abdominal pain, changes in bowel habits, gastrointestinal bleeding, and systemic symptoms of inflammation. Recognition of these signs and symptoms is essential for prompt diagnosis, risk assessment, and initiation of appropriate treatment strategies.

Abdominal Pain

Abdominal pain is the hallmark symptom of diverticular disease and is typically localized to the left lower quadrant (LLQ) of the abdomen, corresponding to the site of diverticular outpouchings in the sigmoid colon. The pain is often described as cramping, intermittent, or colicky in nature and may be exacerbated by eating, defecation, or changes in bowel habits. In diverticulitis, the pain may become more severe and persistent, accompanied by tenderness, guarding, and rebound tenderness on physical examination.

Changes in Bowel Habits

Diverticular disease can cause alterations in bowel habits, including constipation, diarrhea, and alternating patterns of bowel movements. Constipation is a common symptom of diverticulosis, resulting from fecal stasis and colonic motility disorders, whereas diarrhea may occur during acute episodes of diverticulitis or as a consequence of antibiotic therapy. Alternating bowel habits, characterized by periods of constipation and diarrhea, are also common in diverticular disease and may reflect underlying colonic dysmotility.

Gastrointestinal Bleeding

Gastrointestinal bleeding is a common complication of diverticulosis and may manifest as hematochezia (bright red blood per rectum) or melena (dark, tarry stools). Diverticular bleeding typically occurs due to erosion of the mucosal blood vessels overlying the diverticula, leading to brisk or occult bleeding. The severity of bleeding can vary widely, ranging from self-limiting episodes to massive hemorrhage requiring urgent intervention.

Systemic Symptoms of Inflammation

In cases of complicated diverticulitis, systemic symptoms of inflammation may develop, including fever, chills, malaise, and leukocytosis. These systemic symptoms reflect the inflammatory response to colonic infection and inflammation and may accompany local signs of peritonitis, such as rebound tenderness and abdominal guarding. Severe cases of diverticulitis may progress to sepsis, septic shock, or abscess formation, requiring aggressive management and surgical intervention.

Complications of Diverticular Disease

Diverticular disease can lead to various complications, including diverticulitis, abscess formation, perforation, fistula formation, and bowel obstruction. These complications are often associated with severe abdominal pain, systemic symptoms of inflammation, and signs of peritonitis on physical examination. Prompt recognition and management of diverticular disease complications are essential for preventing morbidity and mortality and optimizing patient outcomes.

Chronic Symptoms

In some cases, diverticular disease may present with chronic, recurrent symptoms, such as intermittent abdominal pain, bloating, and changes in bowel habits. These chronic symptoms may be attributed to underlying colonic dysmotility, altered gut-brain axis signaling, and persistent low-grade inflammation. Management of chronic diverticular symptoms often involves dietary modifications, lifestyle interventions, and pharmacological therapy aimed at symptom relief and disease management.

Conclusion

In conclusion, diverticular disease presents with a diverse array of signs and symptoms, reflecting the underlying pathology, disease stage, and individual patient factors. Recognition of these clinical manifestations is essential for accurate diagnosis, risk assessment, and appropriate management of diverticular disease. A comprehensive understanding of the signs and symptoms of diverticular disease is crucial for guiding clinical decision-making, optimizing patient care, and improving outcomes in affected individuals. Further research into the pathophysiology and clinical implications of diverticular disease is warranted to advance our understanding of this common gastrointestinal condition and develop targeted therapeutic interventions.

Navigating the Diagnostic Maze: Differential Diagnosis of Diverticular Disease

Diverticular disease, with its diverse array of signs and symptoms, can pose a diagnostic challenge due to its overlapping clinical presentation with various gastrointestinal and non-gastrointestinal conditions. The differential diagnosis of diverticular disease encompasses a wide range of entities, including inflammatory bowel disease (IBD), colorectal cancer, irritable bowel syndrome (IBS), and urological disorders, among others. Distinguishing between these entities is crucial for accurate diagnosis, appropriate management, and optimal patient care. In this comprehensive analysis, we explore the differential diagnosis of diverticular disease, examining key distinguishing features, diagnostic considerations, and clinical implications associated with each entity.

4.2 Differential Diagnosis

Inflammatory Bowel Disease (IBD)

Inflammatory bowel disease, including Crohn's disease and ulcerative colitis, shares several clinical features with diverticular disease, including abdominal pain, diarrhea, and rectal bleeding. Distinguishing between these entities is essential, as the management and prognosis differ significantly.

- **Key Features**: Inflammatory bowel disease typically presents with a more chronic and relapsing course, with systemic symptoms of inflammation, extraintestinal manifestations, and characteristic endoscopic and histological findings. Crohn's disease may involve any segment of the gastrointestinal tract and is associated with transmural inflammation, skip lesions, and non-caseating granulomas. Ulcerative colitis primarily affects the colon and rectum and is characterized by continuous mucosal inflammation, crypt abscesses, and pseudopolyps.
- **Diagnostic Considerations**: Diagnosis of inflammatory bowel disease relies on a combination of clinical, endoscopic, radiological, and histological findings. Endoscopic evaluation with colonoscopy and biopsy is essential for confirming the diagnosis and distinguishing between Crohn's disease and ulcerative colitis. Radiological imaging, such as computed tomography (CT) or magnetic resonance imaging (MRI), may aid in assessing disease extent and detecting complications, such as strictures, fistulas, and abscesses.
- **Clinical Implications**: Differentiating between diverticular disease and inflammatory bowel disease is crucial for guiding therapeutic

interventions and monitoring disease progression. Treatment of inflammatory bowel disease involves immunosuppressive therapy, biologic agents, and surgical intervention, whereas diverticular disease management focuses on symptom relief, dietary modifications, and preventive strategies aimed at reducing diverticular complications.

Colorectal Cancer

Colorectal cancer shares several clinical features with diverticular disease, including abdominal pain, changes in bowel habits, and rectal bleeding. Distinguishing between these entities is essential, as early detection and treatment of colorectal cancer are associated with improved outcomes.

- **Key Features**: Colorectal cancer often presents with a more insidious onset and progressive course, with symptoms worsening over time. Alarm features, such as unintentional weight loss, anemia, and rectal bleeding, should raise suspicion for colorectal cancer. Endoscopic evaluation with colonoscopy is essential for detecting colorectal neoplasms, including adenomas and carcinomas, and guiding tissue biopsy for histological diagnosis.
- **Diagnostic Considerations**: Diagnosis of colorectal cancer relies on a combination of clinical evaluation, imaging studies, and endoscopic examination. Colonoscopy is the gold standard for colorectal cancer screening and surveillance, allowing for direct visualization of the colonic mucosa and biopsy of suspicious lesions. Radiological imaging, such as CT colonography or MRI, may aid in assessing tumor extent, lymph node involvement, and distant metastases.
- **Clinical Implications**: Early detection and treatment

of colorectal cancer are essential for improving patient outcomes and reducing mortality. Management of colorectal cancer involves a multidisciplinary approach, including surgery, chemotherapy, radiation therapy, and targeted therapy, depending on the stage and extent of disease. Differentiating between diverticular disease and colorectal cancer is crucial for timely intervention and optimal patient care.

Irritable Bowel Syndrome (IBS)

Irritable bowel syndrome shares several clinical features with diverticular disease, including abdominal pain, bloating, and changes in bowel habits. Distinguishing between these entities is essential, as the management and treatment strategies differ significantly.

- **Key Features**: Irritable bowel syndrome is characterized by recurrent abdominal pain or discomfort, associated with alterations in bowel habits, such as diarrhea, constipation, or mixed symptoms. Symptoms may be triggered by stress, dietary factors, or other environmental stimuli. Unlike diverticular disease, irritable bowel syndrome does not typically involve structural abnormalities or inflammatory changes in the colon.
- **Diagnostic Considerations**: Diagnosis of irritable bowel syndrome is based on the Rome IV criteria, which require the presence of recurrent abdominal pain or discomfort, associated with changes in bowel habits, for at least three days per month in the last three months. Diagnostic evaluation may include clinical assessment, symptom diary, and exclusion of other organic gastrointestinal disorders through laboratory tests, imaging studies, and endoscopic examination.

- **Clinical Implications**: Management of irritable bowel syndrome focuses on symptom relief and improving quality of life through dietary modifications, lifestyle interventions, and pharmacological therapy. Psychological interventions, such as cognitive-behavioral therapy and gut-directed hypnotherapy, may also be beneficial in managing symptoms of irritable bowel syndrome. Differentiating between diverticular disease and irritable bowel syndrome is essential for guiding treatment strategies and optimizing patient outcomes.

Urological Disorders

Urological disorders, such as urinary tract infections (UTIs), kidney stones, and bladder dysfunction, may present with symptoms overlapping with diverticular disease, including lower abdominal pain and urinary symptoms. Distinguishing between these entities is essential for accurate diagnosis and appropriate management.

- **Key Features**: Urological disorders often present with symptoms localized to the genitourinary tract, including dysuria, frequency, urgency, hematuria, and suprapubic pain. Lower urinary tract symptoms, such as urinary urgency, frequency, and nocturia, may overlap with symptoms of diverticular disease, leading to diagnostic confusion. In women, gynecological conditions, such as pelvic inflammatory disease (PID) and ovarian cysts, may mimic symptoms of diverticular disease.
- **Diagnostic Considerations**: Diagnosis of urological disorders relies on a combination of clinical evaluation, laboratory tests, imaging studies, and urodynamic assessment. Urinalysis and urine culture are essential for detecting urinary tract infections,

whereas imaging studies, such as ultrasound and CT urography, may aid in diagnosing kidney stones and evaluating bladder function.

- **Clinical Implications:** Prompt recognition and management of urological disorders are essential for preventing complications and optimizing patient outcomes. Treatment of urinary tract infections involves antimicrobial therapy, hydration, and symptomatic relief, whereas management of kidney stones may require medical expulsive therapy or surgical intervention, depending on the size and location of the stone. Differentiating between diverticular disease and urological disorders is crucial for appropriate referral and targeted treatment strategies.

Conclusion

In conclusion, the differential diagnosis of diverticular disease encompasses a wide range of gastrointestinal and non-gastrointestinal conditions, each with its unique clinical features, diagnostic considerations, and management implications. Distinguishing between these entities is essential for accurate diagnosis, appropriate management, and optimal patient care. A comprehensive understanding of the differential diagnosis of diverticular disease is crucial for guiding clinical decision-making, facilitating timely intervention, and improving patient outcomes. Further research into the diagnostic approach and management of diverticular disease and its mimicking conditions is warranted to advance our understanding of this complex clinical entity and enhance patient care.

Exploring Diagnostic Modalities in Diverticular Disease: A Comprehensive Review

Diverticular disease, encompassing diverticulosis and diverticulitis, presents with a spectrum of signs and symptoms that may overlap with various gastrointestinal and non-gastrointestinal conditions. Accurate diagnosis of diverticular disease is essential for guiding appropriate management strategies and optimizing patient outcomes. In this comprehensive review, we explore the diagnostic modalities commonly used in the evaluation of diverticular disease, including colonoscopy, computed tomography (CT) scan, barium enema, and laboratory tests. Each modality offers unique advantages and limitations, and understanding their role in the diagnostic algorithm is crucial for effective clinical decision-making.

4.3 Diagnostic Modalities

Colonoscopy

Colonoscopy is considered the gold standard for the diagnosis of diverticular disease and offers several advantages, including direct visualization of the colonic mucosa, tissue biopsy for histological evaluation, and therapeutic interventions, such as polypectomy and hemostasis.

- **Procedure**: During colonoscopy, a flexible, lighted endoscope is inserted through the rectum and advanced through the entire length of the colon, allowing for direct visualization of the colonic mucosa. The endoscope is equipped with a camera and light

source, enabling real-time imaging of the colonic lumen and identification of diverticular outpouchings.
- **Diagnostic Findings**: Diverticular disease is characterized by the presence of colonic diverticula, small pouch-like protrusions of the colonic wall, typically located in the sigmoid colon. Diverticula appear as small, round or oval-shaped structures, ranging in size from a few millimeters to several centimeters in diameter. The number, size, distribution, and morphology of diverticula are assessed during colonoscopy to determine the severity and extent of diverticular disease.
- **Histological Evaluation**: Tissue biopsy of diverticular mucosa may be performed during colonoscopy to confirm the diagnosis of diverticulosis and exclude other colonic pathologies, such as inflammatory bowel disease (IBD) or colorectal cancer. Histological examination typically reveals nonspecific changes, including mucosal inflammation, fibrosis, and vascular alterations, consistent with diverticular disease.
- **Therapeutic Interventions**: Colonoscopy allows for therapeutic interventions, such as polypectomy, hemostasis, and endoscopic mucosal resection (EMR), in cases of associated colonic polyps, bleeding, or inflammation. Endoscopic management of diverticular bleeding may include hemostatic measures, such as epinephrine injection, thermal coagulation, or endoscopic clipping, depending on the severity and location of bleeding.
- **Limitations**: Despite its utility, colonoscopy has several limitations, including its invasive nature, requirement for bowel preparation, risk of complications, and limited sensitivity for detecting diverticula, particularly in cases of small or flat

lesions. Incomplete visualization of the entire colon may occur due to technical factors, such as poor bowel preparation, inadequate insufflation, or anatomical challenges, leading to missed or overlooked diverticula.

Computed Tomography (CT) Scan

Computed tomography (CT) scan is a valuable imaging modality for the evaluation of diverticular disease, offering high-resolution cross-sectional images of the abdomen and pelvis, detection of diverticula, assessment of complications, and guiding therapeutic interventions.

- **Technique**: CT scan of the abdomen and pelvis is typically performed using a multidetector CT scanner, with intravenous contrast administration to enhance visualization of the colonic wall, mesentery, and surrounding structures. Oral contrast may also be administered to distend the colon and improve delineation of colonic diverticula.
- **Diagnostic Findings**: CT scan allows for the detection and characterization of colonic diverticula, as well as assessment of associated complications, such as diverticulitis, abscess formation, perforation, fistula formation, and bowel obstruction. Diverticula appear as outpouchings of the colonic wall, typically filled with air or fecal material, and may be associated with pericolic fat stranding, inflammatory changes, or fluid collections in cases of diverticulitis.
- **Complication Assessment**: CT scan plays a crucial role in assessing diverticular complications, such as diverticulitis, abscess formation, and perforation, by identifying inflammatory changes, pericolic fat stranding, fluid collections, and free air within the peritoneal cavity. CT imaging helps stratify

the severity of diverticulitis and guide treatment decisions, including the need for antibiotic therapy, percutaneous drainage, or surgical intervention.

- **Therapeutic Guidance**: CT scan may guide therapeutic interventions in cases of complicated diverticulitis, such as percutaneous drainage of abscesses or image-guided placement of colonic stents for bowel obstruction. CT imaging provides detailed anatomical information, allowing for precise localization of pathology and accurate placement of interventional devices.
- **Limitations**: Despite its utility, CT scan has several limitations, including exposure to ionizing radiation, risk of contrast-induced nephropathy, and limited specificity for differentiating between inflammatory and neoplastic colonic lesions. Interpretation of CT images requires expertise in recognizing subtle radiological findings and distinguishing between benign and malignant processes, particularly in cases of colonic wall thickening or mass lesions.

Barium Enema

Barium enema, also known as lower gastrointestinal (GI) series, is a radiographic imaging modality used for the evaluation of diverticular disease, providing detailed visualization of the colonic mucosa, detection of diverticula, and assessment of colonic motility.

- **Procedure**: Barium enema involves the instillation of barium sulfate suspension into the colon through a rectal catheter, followed by fluoroscopic imaging of the colon and rectum. Barium fills the colonic lumen, coating the mucosa and providing contrast for radiographic visualization of colonic morphology and motility.

- **Diagnostic Findings**: Barium enema allows for the detection of colonic diverticula, as well as assessment of diverticular distribution, size, and morphology. Diverticula appear as contrast-filled outpouchings of the colonic wall, typically located in the sigmoid colon, and may demonstrate variable degrees of luminal narrowing or irregularity.
- **Colonic Motility Assessment**: Barium enema provides functional information about colonic motility and transit time by assessing the passage of barium through the colon and rectum. Delayed transit time, segmental hypomotility, or spasmic contractions may be observed in cases of colonic dysmotility, constipation, or diverticular disease.
- **Limitations**: Despite its historical use, barium enema has several limitations, including its invasive nature, requirement for bowel preparation, limited sensitivity for detecting small diverticula, and inability to assess extracolonic structures or complications. The introduction of newer imaging modalities, such as CT scan and magnetic resonance imaging (MRI), has largely replaced barium enema for the evaluation of diverticular disease due to their superior sensitivity and specificity.

Laboratory Tests

Laboratory tests play a supportive role in the diagnosis and management of diverticular disease, providing valuable information about inflammatory markers, infection, anemia, and electrolyte abnormalities.

- **Complete Blood Count (CBC)**: CBC may reveal leukocytosis, indicative of systemic inflammation or infection, and anemia, secondary to gastrointestinal bleeding or chronic disease. Elevated white blood cell (WBC) count and left shift may suggest acute diverticulitis, whereas microcytic anemia may indicate chronic bleeding from diverticular disease.

- **Inflammatory Markers**: Serum inflammatory markers, such as C-reactive protein (CRP) and erythrocyte sedimentation rate (ESR), are commonly elevated in cases of diverticulitis, reflecting the presence of inflammation and tissue injury. Elevated CRP and ESR levels correlate with disease severity and response to treatment and may aid in monitoring disease activity and guiding therapeutic decisions.
- **Stool Studies**: Stool studies, including fecal occult blood test (FOBT) and fecal calprotectin assay, may be performed to detect occult blood and assess intestinal inflammation in patients with diverticular disease. Positive FOBT may indicate active gastrointestinal bleeding, whereas elevated fecal calprotectin levels suggest mucosal inflammation and may predict disease recurrence or complications.
- **Electrolyte and Renal Function Tests**: Electrolyte and renal function tests may be performed to assess for electrolyte abnormalities, dehydration, or renal insufficiency in patients with diverticular disease, particularly during acute exacerbations or complications. Serum electrolyte imbalances, such as hypokalemia or hyponatremia, may occur secondary to vomiting, diarrhea, or fluid loss, whereas acute kidney injury may result from sepsis, dehydration, or contrast nephropathy.
- **Limitations**: Although laboratory tests provide valuable diagnostic information, they lack specificity for diverticular disease and may be influenced by various factors, such as concurrent infections, medications, or comorbidities. Interpretation of laboratory results should be correlated with clinical

findings and imaging studies to establish an accurate diagnosis and guide appropriate management.

Conclusion

In conclusion, a multidisciplinary approach incorporating various diagnostic modalities is essential for the accurate diagnosis and management of diverticular disease. Colonoscopy remains the gold standard for the evaluation of diverticulosis and diverticulitis, providing direct visualization of colonic mucosa and tissue biopsy for histological assessment. Computed tomography (CT) scan offers high-resolution imaging of the abdomen and pelvis, allowing for the detection of diverticular disease, assessment of complications, and guiding therapeutic interventions. Barium enema provides functional information about colonic motility and transit time, although its use has largely been supplanted by newer imaging modalities. Laboratory tests play a supportive role in the diagnosis and management of diverticular disease, providing valuable information about inflammatory markers, infection, anemia, and electrolyte abnormalities. A comprehensive understanding of these diagnostic modalities and their respective strengths and limitations is crucial for effective clinical decision-making and optimizing patient outcomes in diverticular disease. Further research into novel diagnostic approaches and biomarkers may enhance our ability to diagnose, risk-stratify, and manage diverticular disease more effectively in the future.

CHAPTER 5: COMPLICATIONS OF DIVERTICULOSIS

Navigating the Landscape of Diverticulitis: Understanding Classification, Grading, and Pathophysiology

Diverticulitis, a common inflammatory condition of the colon, poses significant challenges in diagnosis, management, and prevention. This section explores the classification and grading systems used to stratify diverticulitis severity, as well as the intricate pathophysiological mechanisms underlying its development and progression.

5.1 Diverticulitis

Classification and Grading

Diverticulitis classification and grading systems serve as essential tools for stratifying disease severity, guiding treatment decisions, and predicting patient outcomes. Several classification systems have been proposed, each incorporating clinical, radiological, and endoscopic findings to categorize diverticulitis into various stages of severity.

- **Hinchey Classification:** The Hinchey classification, initially proposed in 1978 and subsequently modified, categorizes diverticulitis based on the presence and extent of intra-abdominal abscesses, fecal peritonitis, and purulent or fecal peritonitis. The four stages of Hinchey classification include:
    - Stage I: Pericolic abscess
    - Stage II: Pelvic, retroperitoneal, or distant abscess
    - Stage III: Fecal peritonitis
    - Stage IV: Generalized purulent or fecal peritonitis
- **Ambrosetti Classification:** The Ambrosetti classification, introduced in 2000, expands upon the Hinchey classification by incorporating radiological findings and treatment options. The Ambrosetti classification includes four stages:
    - Stage 0: Uncomplicated diverticulitis
    - Stage I: Confined abscess or phlegmon
    - Stage II: Extraluminal air or free perforation
    - Stage III: Diffuse peritonitis
- **Modified Hinchey Classification:** The modified Hinchey classification, proposed in 2004, incorporates both clinical and radiological criteria to classify diverticulitis severity and guide treatment decisions. The modified Hinchey classification includes:
    - Stage 0: Uncomplicated diverticulitis
    - Stage Ia: Confined pericolic inflammation or small abscess
    - Stage Ib: Larger abscess requiring percutaneous drainage
    - Stage II: Pelvic, retroperitoneal, or distant abscess
    - Stage III: Generalized purulent peritonitis
    - Stage IV: Fecal peritonitis

Grading systems complement classification schemes by assigning a severity grade to diverticulitis based on clinical, laboratory, and imaging parameters. Grading systems help assess disease severity, predict treatment response, and guide surgical decision-making. The severity of diverticulitis is graded based on the presence and extent of inflammation, abscess formation, peritonitis, and associated complications.

Pathophysiology of Diverticulitis

The pathophysiology of diverticulitis is multifactorial, involving complex interactions between genetic, environmental, dietary, microbiological, and inflammatory factors. Several mechanisms contribute to diverticulitis development and progression, including colonic wall weakness, luminal obstruction, bacterial overgrowth, mucosal injury, and immune dysregulation.

- **Colonic Wall Weakness**: Diverticulitis often arises from colonic wall weakness, predisposing to diverticular outpouching formation and subsequent inflammation. Colonic wall weakness may result from structural alterations, such as smooth muscle hypertrophy, collagen deposition, and elastin degradation, leading to focal areas of weakness and herniation of the mucosal and submucosal layers.
- **Luminal Obstruction**: Luminal obstruction plays a crucial role in diverticulitis pathogenesis by promoting stasis, bacterial overgrowth, and mucosal injury. Fecal material, undigested food particles, and gas accumulate within diverticula, creating an anaerobic environment conducive to bacterial proliferation and fermentation. Luminal obstruction may be exacerbated by dietary factors, such as low-fiber diets, inadequate fluid intake, and altered colonic motility patterns.
- **Bacterial Overgrowth**: Bacterial overgrowth within

diverticula leads to microbial fermentation, gas production, and local inflammation, contributing to diverticulitis pathogenesis. The colonic microbiota undergo dysbiosis in diverticular disease, with shifts in microbial composition, diversity, and metabolic activity. Pathogenic bacteria, such as Enterobacteriaceae, Bacteroides, and Clostridium species, may proliferate within diverticula, leading to mucosal injury, inflammation, and infection.

- **Mucosal Injury**: Mucosal injury and inflammation occur as a consequence of luminal obstruction, bacterial overgrowth, and immune activation. Increased luminal pressure within diverticula leads to mucosal stretching, ischemia, and microperforation, predisposing to mucosal injury and breach of the mucosal barrier. Mucosal injury triggers an inflammatory response, characterized by leukocyte recruitment, cytokine release, and tissue remodeling, leading to acute inflammation and abscess formation.
- **Immune Dysregulation**: Immune dysregulation plays a central role in diverticulitis pathophysiology, contributing to aberrant inflammatory responses, impaired mucosal immunity, and chronic inflammation. Genetic factors, such as polymorphisms in inflammatory cytokine genes, may predispose individuals to immune dysregulation and exaggerated inflammatory responses. Dysregulated immune responses may lead to recurrent diverticulitis episodes, chronic inflammation, and disease progression.

Understanding the pathophysiological mechanisms underlying diverticulitis is essential for developing targeted therapeutic interventions aimed at preventing disease onset, reducing inflammation, and preventing disease recurrence. Further research into the genetic, environmental, and microbial factors contributing to diverticulitis pathogenesis is warranted to advance our understanding of this common gastrointestinal condition and develop more effective treatment strategies.

Unraveling the Complexity of Abscess Formation in Diverticulitis: Insights and Implications

Abscess formation represents a common complication of diverticulitis, characterized by the localized accumulation of purulent material within the pericolonic or intra-abdominal space. This section delves into the multifaceted process of abscess formation in diverticulitis, exploring the underlying pathophysiological mechanisms, clinical manifestations, diagnostic considerations, and therapeutic implications.

5.2 Abscess Formation

Abscess formation in diverticulitis arises from a cascade of events initiated by colonic wall inflammation, bacterial proliferation, and tissue injury. The complex interplay between microbial factors, host immune responses, and anatomical considerations contributes to abscess development, progression, and clinical sequelae.

Pathophysiological Mechanisms

The pathophysiological mechanisms underlying abscess formation in diverticulitis involve a series of interconnected events, including:

- **Colonic Wall Inflammation**: Diverticulitis begins with inflammation of the colonic wall, triggered by luminal obstruction, bacterial overgrowth, and mucosal injury. Inflammatory mediators, such as cytokines, chemokines, and reactive oxygen species, recruit

leukocytes to the site of injury, initiating an immune response and tissue remodeling.
- **Microbial Factors**: Bacterial overgrowth within diverticula leads to microbial fermentation, gas production, and local inflammation. Pathogenic bacteria, such as Escherichia coli, Bacteroides fragilis, and Enterococcus species, proliferate within diverticula, releasing toxins and inflammatory molecules that exacerbate tissue injury and inflammation.
- **Tissue Injury and Necrosis**: Prolonged inflammation and bacterial proliferation lead to tissue injury, necrosis, and breakdown of the mucosal barrier. Microperforations within diverticula allow the escape of luminal contents into the pericolonic or intra-abdominal space, triggering an inflammatory response and abscess formation.
- **Anatomical Considerations**: Anatomical factors, such as diverticular location, size, and morphology, influence the likelihood of abscess formation and clinical outcomes. Diverticula located in the sigmoid colon are more prone to abscess formation due to higher luminal pressures and increased bacterial burden. Large or complex diverticula may harbor greater quantities of fecal material and bacteria, predisposing to abscess development.

Clinical Manifestations

Abscess formation in diverticulitis presents with a spectrum of clinical manifestations, including:

- **Localized Pain**: Abscesses typically manifest as localized abdominal or pelvic pain, often described as sharp, constant, or throbbing in nature. The pain may be exacerbated by movement, palpation,

or changes in position and is often associated with tenderness, guarding, or rebound tenderness on physical examination.
- **Systemic Symptoms**: Systemic symptoms of inflammation, such as fever, chills, malaise, and leukocytosis, may accompany abscess formation in diverticulitis. Elevated inflammatory markers, such as C-reactive protein (CRP) and erythrocyte sedimentation rate (ESR), may be observed, reflecting the severity of inflammation and tissue injury.
- **Altered Bowel Habits**: Abscess formation may disrupt normal bowel habits, leading to changes in stool frequency, consistency, and caliber. Patients may experience constipation, diarrhea, or alternating patterns of bowel movements, reflecting underlying colonic inflammation and dysmotility.
- **Peritoneal Signs**: Severe cases of abscess formation may present with signs of peritonitis, such as rebound tenderness, abdominal distension, and rigidity. Peritoneal signs indicate the presence of diffuse inflammation and infection within the peritoneal cavity, requiring urgent intervention and surgical evaluation.

Diagnostic Considerations

The diagnosis of abscess formation in diverticulitis relies on a combination of clinical evaluation, laboratory tests, and imaging studies, including:

- **Clinical Assessment**: Clinical evaluation includes history taking, physical examination, and assessment of vital signs. Localized abdominal or pelvic pain, tenderness, and systemic symptoms of inflammation may raise suspicion for abscess formation and prompt further diagnostic evaluation.

- **Laboratory Tests**: Laboratory tests, such as complete blood count (CBC) and inflammatory markers (e.g., CRP, ESR), provide valuable information about systemic inflammation, infection, and leukocyte response. Elevated white blood cell (WBC) count and inflammatory markers may indicate abscess formation and guide treatment decisions.
- **Imaging Studies**: Imaging studies, such as computed tomography (CT) scan and ultrasound, play a crucial role in the diagnosis and characterization of abscesses in diverticulitis. CT scan offers high-resolution cross-sectional images of the abdomen and pelvis, allowing for the detection of abscesses, assessment of size, location, and associated complications.

Therapeutic Implications

The management of abscess formation in diverticulitis involves a multidisciplinary approach, including medical therapy, percutaneous drainage, and surgical intervention, depending on abscess size, location, and clinical stability.

- **Medical Therapy**: Initial management of abscess formation may include broad-spectrum antibiotics to cover enteric pathogens and anaerobic bacteria. Antibiotic therapy should be guided by culture and sensitivity results and continued until resolution of clinical symptoms and normalization of inflammatory markers.
- **Percutaneous Drainage**: Percutaneous drainage of abscesses is a minimally invasive procedure performed under imaging guidance, such as ultrasound or CT, to evacuate purulent material and decompress the abscess cavity. Percutaneous drainage is indicated for large, symptomatic abscesses or those associated with systemic symptoms of inflammation.

- **Surgical Intervention**: Surgical intervention may be required for complicated abscesses, such as those refractory to percutaneous drainage, associated with bowel perforation, or complicated by sepsis. Surgical options include laparoscopic or open surgical drainage, segmental resection of the affected colon, or Hartmann's procedure in cases of severe disease or hemodynamic instability.

Conclusion

In conclusion, abscess formation represents a common and potentially serious complication of diverticulitis, characterized by localized purulent collection within the pericolonic or intra-abdominal space. The pathophysiology of abscess formation involves a complex interplay between colonic wall inflammation, bacterial proliferation, tissue injury, and host immune responses. Clinical manifestations of abscess formation include localized pain, systemic symptoms of inflammation, altered bowel habits, and peritoneal signs. Diagnostic evaluation of abscesses in diverticulitis relies on clinical assessment, laboratory tests, and imaging studies, with CT scan serving as the gold standard for abscess detection and characterization. Management of abscess formation involves a multidisciplinary approach, including medical therapy, percutaneous drainage, and surgical intervention, tailored to abscess size, location, and clinical stability. Further research into the pathophysiology, diagnosis, and management of abscess formation in diverticulitis is warranted to optimize patient outcomes and reduce the burden of this common gastrointestinal condition.

Exploring Perforation and Peritonitis in Diverticulitis: A Comprehensive Analysis

Perforation and peritonitis represent severe and potentially life-threatening complications of diverticulitis, posing significant diagnostic and therapeutic challenges. This section provides a thorough examination of perforation and peritonitis in the context of diverticulitis, encompassing their pathophysiology, clinical manifestations, diagnostic considerations, and therapeutic interventions.

5.3 Perforation and Peritonitis

Perforation and peritonitis in diverticulitis arise from the breach of the colonic wall and spillage of luminal contents into the peritoneal cavity, triggering an inflammatory response and systemic sepsis. Understanding the underlying mechanisms and clinical implications of perforation and peritonitis is essential for timely diagnosis and appropriate management.

Pathophysiology

The pathophysiology of perforation and peritonitis in diverticulitis involves a cascade of events, including:

- **Colonic Wall Weakness**: Diverticulitis often originates from colonic wall weakness, predisposing to diverticular outpouching formation and subsequent perforation. Structural alterations, such as smooth muscle hypertrophy, collagen deposition, and elastin degradation, weaken the colonic wall, increasing susceptibility to perforation under conditions of luminal obstruction and inflammation.

- **Microbial Overgrowth**: Bacterial overgrowth within diverticula leads to microbial fermentation, gas production, and local inflammation. Pathogenic bacteria, such as Escherichia coli, Bacteroides fragilis, and Enterococcus species, proliferate within diverticula, releasing toxins and inflammatory molecules that exacerbate tissue injury and inflammation.
- **Mucosal Injury and Microperforation**: Prolonged inflammation and bacterial proliferation result in mucosal injury, necrosis, and breakdown of the mucosal barrier. Microperforations within diverticula allow the escape of luminal contents, including fecal material, bacteria, and inflammatory mediators, into the peritoneal cavity, initiating an inflammatory cascade and peritoneal response.
- **Peritoneal Inflammation and Sepsis**: Perforation of the colonic wall triggers an inflammatory response within the peritoneal cavity, characterized by leukocyte recruitment, cytokine release, and vascular permeability. Peritoneal inflammation leads to the formation of exudates, adhesions, and abscesses, contributing to systemic sepsis, multiorgan dysfunction, and septic shock.

Clinical Manifestations

Perforation and peritonitis in diverticulitis present with a constellation of clinical manifestations, including:

- **Acute Abdominal Pain**: Perforation and peritonitis typically manifest as sudden-onset, severe, and diffuse abdominal pain, often described as sharp, stabbing, or constant in nature. The pain may be aggravated by movement, palpation, or changes in position and is often associated with guarding, rigidity, and rebound

tenderness on physical examination.
- **Systemic Symptoms of Sepsis**: Perforation and peritonitis may lead to systemic sepsis, characterized by fever, chills, tachycardia, hypotension, and altered mental status. Systemic symptoms of sepsis reflect the severity of inflammation, bacterial dissemination, and host response, requiring urgent medical intervention and supportive care.
- **Gastrointestinal Symptoms**: Gastrointestinal symptoms, such as nausea, vomiting, anorexia, and diarrhea, may accompany perforation and peritonitis, reflecting underlying colonic inflammation, dysmotility, and disruption of normal bowel function.
- **Peritoneal Signs**: Severe cases of perforation and peritonitis may present with signs of peritoneal irritation, such as rebound tenderness, abdominal distension, and absent bowel sounds. Peritoneal signs indicate the presence of diffuse inflammation and infection within the peritoneal cavity, requiring urgent surgical evaluation and intervention.

Diagnostic Considerations

The diagnosis of perforation and peritonitis in diverticulitis relies on a combination of clinical evaluation, laboratory tests, and imaging studies, including:

- **Clinical Assessment**: Clinical evaluation includes history taking, physical examination, and assessment of vital signs. Acute onset of severe abdominal pain, systemic symptoms of sepsis, and peritoneal signs should raise suspicion for perforation and peritonitis and prompt further diagnostic evaluation.
- **Laboratory Tests**: Laboratory tests, such as complete blood count (CBC), inflammatory markers (e.g., C-reactive protein, erythrocyte sedimentation

rate), and serum electrolytes, provide valuable information about systemic inflammation, infection, and metabolic derangements. Elevated white blood cell (WBC) count, bandemia, and metabolic acidosis may indicate severe sepsis and multiorgan dysfunction.
- **Imaging Studies**: Imaging studies, such as computed tomography (CT) scan and abdominal ultrasound, play a crucial role in the diagnosis and characterization of perforation and peritonitis. CT scan offers high-resolution cross-sectional images of the abdomen and pelvis, allowing for the detection of free air, fluid collections, and peritoneal inflammation associated with perforation and peritonitis.

Therapeutic Interventions

The management of perforation and peritonitis in diverticulitis involves a multidisciplinary approach, including medical therapy, fluid resuscitation, antibiotics, and surgical intervention, depending on clinical stability, severity of sepsis, and extent of peritoneal contamination.

- **Medical Therapy**: Initial management of perforation and peritonitis may include aggressive fluid resuscitation, broad-spectrum antibiotics, and supportive care in the intensive care unit (ICU). Antibiotic therapy should cover enteric pathogens and anaerobic bacteria and be guided by culture and sensitivity results.
- **Surgical Intervention**: Surgical intervention is indicated for complicated cases of perforation and peritonitis, such as those refractory to medical therapy, associated with septic shock, or complicated by intra-abdominal abscesses. Surgical options include exploratory laparotomy, peritoneal lavage, segmental resection of the affected colon, and creation of a

diverting colostomy or Hartmann's procedure.

Conclusion

In conclusion, perforation and peritonitis represent severe and potentially life-threatening complications of diverticulitis, characterized by the breach of the colonic wall and spillage of luminal contents into the peritoneal cavity. The pathophysiology of perforation and peritonitis involves colonic wall weakness, microbial overgrowth, mucosal injury, and peritoneal inflammation, leading to systemic sepsis and multiorgan dysfunction. Clinical manifestations of perforation and peritonitis include acute abdominal pain, systemic symptoms of sepsis, gastrointestinal symptoms, and peritoneal signs. Diagnostic evaluation relies on clinical assessment, laboratory tests, and imaging studies, with CT scan serving as the gold standard for perforation and peritonitis detection. Management involves a multidisciplinary approach, including medical therapy, fluid resuscitation, antibiotics, and surgical intervention, tailored to clinical stability, severity of sepsis, and extent of peritoneal contamination. Further research into the pathophysiology, diagnosis, and management of perforation and peritonitis in diverticulitis is warranted to improve patient outcomes and reduce the morbidity and mortality associated with these serious complications.

Exploring Fistula Formation in Diverticulitis: Understanding Pathogenesis, Clinical Implications, and Management Strategies

Fistula formation represents a significant complication of diverticulitis, characterized by the abnormal communication between two epithelial-lined surfaces, such as the colon and adjacent structures. This section provides a comprehensive analysis of fistula formation in diverticulitis, encompassing its pathophysiology, clinical manifestations, diagnostic considerations, and therapeutic interventions.

5.4 Fistula Formation

Fistula formation in diverticulitis arises from the inflammatory process involving adjacent structures, leading to erosion, necrosis, and eventual perforation. The complex interplay between colonic inflammation, tissue injury, and adjacent organ involvement contributes to fistula development, progression, and clinical sequelae.

Pathophysiology

The pathophysiology of fistula formation in diverticulitis involves several key mechanisms:

- **Colonic Inflammation**: Diverticulitis is characterized by inflammation of the colonic wall, triggered by luminal obstruction, bacterial overgrowth, and mucosal injury. Inflammatory mediators, such as cytokines and chemokines, recruit leukocytes to the site of injury, leading to tissue edema, necrosis, and ulceration.
- **Adjacent Organ Involvement**: In severe cases of diverticulitis, inflammation may extend beyond the colonic wall to involve adjacent structures, such as the bladder, small bowel, or pelvic organs. Continued inflammation and tissue necrosis predispose to adhesion formation, tissue fusion, and eventual fistula tract formation.
- **Erosion and Perforation**: Prolonged inflammation and tissue injury result in erosion, necrosis, and breakdown of the colonic mucosa, leading to microperforations and breach of the mucosal

barrier. Luminal contents, including fecal material, bacteria, and inflammatory exudates, escape into the peritoneal cavity or adjacent structures, initiating an inflammatory cascade and fistula formation.

- **Fistula Tract Formation**: Fistula formation occurs as a result of the aberrant healing process, characterized by granulation tissue formation, fibrosis, and epithelialization along the tract. Persistent inflammation and bacterial colonization perpetuate fistula tract formation, leading to chronic infection, drainage, and clinical symptoms.

Clinical Manifestations

Fistula formation in diverticulitis presents with a variety of clinical manifestations, depending on the location and extent of the fistula tract:

- **Enterocolonic Fistulas**: Enterocolonic fistulas, involving communication between the colon and adjacent bowel segments, may present with symptoms of fecal urgency, diarrhea, hematochezia, or passage of gas or stool through the vagina or urethra (enterovesical, enterovaginal, or enterourethral fistulas).
- **Colovesical Fistulas**: Colovesical fistulas, connecting the colon and urinary bladder, may manifest as pneumaturia, fecaluria, recurrent urinary tract infections (UTIs), or passage of gas or stool through the urethra during defecation.
- **Colovaginal Fistulas**: Colovaginal fistulas, linking the colon and vagina, may present with symptoms of fecal or gas passage through the vagina, recurrent vaginal infections, or foul-smelling vaginal discharge.
- **Colouterine Fistulas**: Colouterine fistulas, connecting the colon and uterus, may present with symptoms

of cyclic hematochezia coinciding with menstruation, foul-smelling vaginal discharge, or pelvic pain.
- **Perianal Fistulas**: Perianal fistulas, extending from the anal canal to the perianal skin or adjacent structures, may present with symptoms of perianal discharge, pain, swelling, or recurrent abscess formation.

Diagnostic Considerations

The diagnosis of fistula formation in diverticulitis relies on a combination of clinical evaluation, imaging studies, and endoscopic evaluation:

- **Clinical Assessment**: Clinical evaluation includes history taking, physical examination, and assessment of symptoms suggestive of fistula formation, such as fecal or gas passage through non-anal routes, recurrent UTIs, or perianal discharge.
- **Imaging Studies**: Imaging studies, such as computed tomography (CT) scan, magnetic resonance imaging (MRI), or contrast-enhanced studies (e.g., barium enema, cystography), play a crucial role in the diagnosis and characterization of fistulas. CT scan offers high-resolution cross-sectional images of the abdomen and pelvis, allowing for the detection of fistula tracts, associated complications, and adjacent organ involvement.
- **Endoscopic Evaluation**: Endoscopic evaluation, including colonoscopy or flexible sigmoidoscopy, may be performed to directly visualize the colonic mucosa, identify diverticula, and assess for fistula openings or mucosal abnormalities. Endoscopic retrograde cholangiopancreatography (ERCP) may be indicated for suspected biliary-enteric fistulas or pancreatic-enteric fistulas.

Therapeutic Interventions

The management of fistula formation in diverticulitis involves a multidisciplinary approach, including medical therapy, minimally invasive procedures, and surgical intervention:

- **Medical Therapy**: Initial management of fistula formation may include conservative measures, such as antibiotics, bowel rest, and symptom management. Antibiotic therapy should cover enteric pathogens and anaerobic bacteria, guided by culture and sensitivity results.
- **Minimally Invasive Procedures**: Minimally invasive techniques, such as endoscopic stent placement, fibrin glue injection, or collagen plug insertion, may be considered for selected cases of fistula formation, particularly those amenable to less invasive interventions and with minimal associated morbidity.
- **Surgical Intervention**: Surgical intervention is indicated for complicated or refractory cases of fistula formation, such as those associated with abscesses, strictures, or significant tissue involvement. Surgical options include fistula excision, segmental resection of the affected colon, and primary anastomosis with or without diversion.

Conclusion

In conclusion, fistula formation represents a significant complication of diverticulitis, characterized by abnormal communication between the colon and adjacent structures. The pathophysiology of fistula formation involves colonic inflammation, tissue injury, adjacent organ involvement, and aberrant healing processes. Clinical manifestations of fistula formation vary depending on the location and extent of the fistula tract, ranging from fecal or gas passage through non-anal routes to recurrent UTIs or perianal discharge. Diagnostic evaluation relies on a combination of clinical assessment, imaging studies, and endoscopic evaluation, with CT scan serving as the gold standard for fistula detection and characterization. Management involves a multidisciplinary approach, including medical therapy, minimally invasive procedures, and surgical intervention, tailored to individual patient characteristics and clinical presentation. Further research into the pathophysiology, diagnosis, and management of fistula formation in diverticulitis is warranted to optimize patient outcomes and reduce the morbidity associated with this challenging complication.

Navigating Obstruction in Diverticulitis: Understanding Mechanisms, Clinical Features, and Management Strategies

Obstruction represents a significant complication of diverticulitis, contributing to bowel dysfunction, abdominal pain, and potential surgical intervention. This section provides a comprehensive exploration of obstruction in diverticulitis, encompassing its pathophysiology, clinical manifestations, diagnostic considerations, and therapeutic interventions.

5.5 Obstruction

Obstruction in diverticulitis arises from luminal narrowing, stricture formation, or mechanical obstruction secondary to inflammatory processes, leading to impaired bowel transit and functional impairment. Understanding the underlying mechanisms and clinical implications of obstruction is crucial for timely diagnosis and appropriate management.

Pathophysiology

The pathophysiology of obstruction in diverticulitis involves several key mechanisms:

- **Luminal Narrowing**: Chronic inflammation and fibrosis within the colonic wall may lead to luminal narrowing or stricture formation, restricting the passage of stool and gas. Luminal narrowing may result from repeated episodes of diverticulitis, tissue scarring, or healing processes following acute inflammation.
- **Mechanical Obstruction**: Acute inflammation, abscess formation, or fecal impaction within diverticula may cause mechanical obstruction, preventing the passage of luminal contents and leading to bowel distension and functional impairment. Mechanical obstruction may be exacerbated by luminal edema, adhesions, or external compression from adjacent structures.
- **Functional Impairment**: Obstruction in diverticulitis results in functional impairment of colonic motility, leading to symptoms of bowel obstruction, such as abdominal distension, crampy abdominal pain, nausea, vomiting, and constipation. Functional impairment may predispose to bacterial overgrowth, fecal stasis, and exacerbation of inflammation.

Clinical Manifestations

Obstruction in diverticulitis presents with a variety of clinical manifestations, depending on the location, severity, and duration of obstruction:

- **Abdominal Distension**: Obstruction may lead to abdominal distension, bloating, and discomfort, reflecting bowel dilation and functional impairment. Abdominal distension may be accompanied by

tympany on percussion and hypoactive or absent bowel sounds on auscultation.
- **Crampy Abdominal Pain**: Patients may experience crampy abdominal pain, often localized to the lower abdomen or left iliac fossa, exacerbated by meals and relieved by bowel movements. Abdominal pain may be associated with nausea, vomiting, and anorexia.
- **Altered Bowel Habits**: Obstruction may result in altered bowel habits, such as constipation, diarrhea, or alternating patterns of bowel movements. Patients may experience difficulty passing stool or gas, leading to straining, incomplete evacuation, and abdominal discomfort.
- **Systemic Symptoms**: Severe cases of obstruction may present with systemic symptoms of dehydration, electrolyte imbalance, and metabolic derangements, requiring urgent medical intervention and fluid resuscitation.

Diagnostic Considerations

The diagnosis of obstruction in diverticulitis relies on a combination of clinical evaluation, imaging studies, and laboratory tests:

- **Clinical Assessment**: Clinical evaluation includes history taking, physical examination, and assessment of symptoms suggestive of obstruction, such as abdominal distension, crampy abdominal pain, nausea, vomiting, and altered bowel habits.
- **Imaging Studies**: Imaging studies, such as abdominal X-ray, computed tomography (CT) scan, or barium enema, play a crucial role in the diagnosis and characterization of obstruction. Abdominal X-ray may reveal signs of bowel distension, air-fluid levels, or fecal impaction, whereas CT scan offers high-

resolution images of the abdomen and pelvis, allowing for the detection of obstructive lesions, stricture formation, or colonic dilatation.
- **Laboratory Tests**: Laboratory tests, such as complete blood count (CBC), electrolyte panel, and inflammatory markers (e.g., C-reactive protein, erythrocyte sedimentation rate), provide valuable information about systemic inflammation, infection, and metabolic status. Elevated white blood cell (WBC) count, bandemia, and electrolyte abnormalities may indicate severe obstruction or associated complications.

Therapeutic Interventions

The management of obstruction in diverticulitis involves a stepwise approach, including conservative measures, bowel decompression, and surgical intervention, depending on the severity, duration, and underlying etiology of obstruction:

- **Conservative Measures**: Initial management of obstruction may include bowel rest, intravenous fluids, electrolyte replacement, and symptomatic relief with antiemetics and analgesics. Dietary modifications, such as a low-residue or clear liquid diet, may be implemented to reduce colonic workload and promote bowel rest.
- **Bowel Decompression**: Bowel decompression may be achieved through nasogastric or rectal tube placement, aiming to relieve colonic distension, decompress gas and stool, and alleviate symptoms of obstruction. Bowel decompression is typically reserved for acute, uncomplicated cases of obstruction and may be performed in conjunction with conservative measures.
- **Surgical Intervention**: Surgical intervention is

indicated for refractory or complicated cases of obstruction, such as those associated with complete bowel obstruction, ischemia, perforation, or peritonitis. Surgical options include segmental resection of the affected colon, primary anastomosis with or without diversion, or creation of a diverting colostomy or ileostomy.

Conclusion

In conclusion, obstruction represents a significant complication of diverticulitis, characterized by luminal narrowing, stricture formation, or mechanical obstruction secondary to inflammatory processes. The pathophysiology of obstruction involves luminal narrowing, mechanical obstruction, and functional impairment of colonic motility, leading to abdominal distension, crampy abdominal pain, altered bowel habits, and systemic symptoms. Diagnostic evaluation relies on clinical assessment, imaging studies, and laboratory tests, with CT scan serving as the gold standard for obstruction detection and characterization. Management involves a stepwise approach, including conservative measures, bowel decompression, and surgical intervention, tailored to individual patient characteristics and clinical presentation. Further research into the pathophysiology, diagnosis, and management of obstruction in diverticulitis is warranted to optimize patient outcomes and reduce the morbidity associated with this challenging complication.

CHAPTER 6: MEDICAL MANAGEMENT OF DIVERTICULOSIS

6.1 Conservative Management: Navigating Dietary Modifications and Pharmacotherapy in Diverticulitis

Diverticulitis often necessitates a multifaceted approach to management, with conservative measures playing a pivotal role in alleviating symptoms, promoting healing, and preventing disease recurrence. This section delves into the intricacies of conservative management, focusing on dietary modifications and pharmacotherapy as cornerstone interventions in the management of diverticulitis.

Conservative Management

Conservative management encompasses a spectrum of non-invasive strategies aimed at symptom control, reduction of inflammation, and restoration of colonic health. While surgical intervention may be required in severe or refractory cases, conservative measures form the foundation of initial treatment and long-term management in diverticulitis.

Dietary Modifications

Dietary modifications represent a cornerstone of conservative management in diverticulitis, aimed at reducing colonic irritation, promoting regular bowel movements, and preventing exacerbations of inflammation. Several dietary approaches have been proposed, each with unique benefits and considerations:

High-Fiber Diet: A high-fiber diet is commonly recommended for individuals with diverticulitis, as it helps maintain bowel regularity, promote stool bulk, and prevent fecal stasis within diverticula. Fiber-rich foods, such as fruits, vegetables, whole grains, and legumes, contain insoluble and soluble fiber components that facilitate smooth bowel transit and minimize straining during defecation. Adequate fiber intake has been associated with reduced risk of diverticulitis development and recurrence, making it a cornerstone of dietary management. However, it's important to introduce fiber gradually and ensure adequate hydration to prevent bloating, gas, and discomfort.

Low-FODMAP Diet: Some individuals with diverticulitis may experience symptoms related to fermentable carbohydrates, such as fructans, oligosaccharides, disaccharides, monosaccharides, and polyols (FODMAPs). In such cases, a low-FODMAP diet may be beneficial in reducing symptoms of bloating, gas, and abdominal discomfort. This diet restricts high-FODMAP foods, such as certain fruits (e.g., apples, pears), vegetables (e.g., onions, garlic), dairy products (e.g., milk, soft cheeses), legumes, and sweeteners, while promoting low-FODMAP alternatives. However, long-term adherence to a low-FODMAP diet should be supervised by a healthcare professional to ensure nutritional adequacy and prevent dietary deficiencies.

Clear Liquid Diet: During acute exacerbations of diverticulitis, a clear liquid diet may be recommended to provide bowel rest, alleviate symptoms, and minimize colonic workload. Clear liquids, such as broth, clear soups, fruit juices (without pulp), gelatin, and clear sports drinks, are easily digestible and leave minimal residue in the colon. A clear liquid diet should be temporary and followed by gradual reintroduction of solid foods as tolerated.

Low-Residue Diet: A low-residue diet may be prescribed during acute exacerbations or periods of bowel rest in diverticulitis, aiming to reduce fecal bulk, minimize bowel irritation, and alleviate symptoms of abdominal pain and cramping. This diet restricts high-residue foods, such as whole grains, raw fruits and vegetables, nuts, seeds, and fibrous foods, while emphasizing low-residue alternatives, such as white rice, refined grains, cooked fruits and vegetables (without skins or seeds), and lean proteins. However, long-term adherence to a low-residue diet should be balanced with the need for adequate fiber intake to prevent constipation and maintain colonic health.

Pharmacotherapy

Pharmacotherapy plays a crucial role in the management of diverticulitis, targeting inflammation, pain, infection, and symptomatic relief. Pharmacological agents are often used in conjunction with dietary modifications and lifestyle interventions to achieve optimal outcomes:

Antibiotics: Antibiotics are commonly prescribed in acute episodes of diverticulitis to eradicate bacterial overgrowth, reduce inflammation, and prevent disease progression. Empiric antibiotic therapy typically covers enteric pathogens and anaerobic bacteria, with regimens such as ciprofloxacin and metronidazole, or amoxicillin-clavulanate. The duration and choice of antibiotics depend on disease severity, clinical response, and microbiological findings. However, the routine use of antibiotics in uncomplicated diverticulitis is debated, with growing emphasis on selective antibiotic use to minimize antibiotic resistance and adverse effects.

Analgesics: Analgesic agents, such as nonsteroidal anti-inflammatory drugs (NSAIDs) and acetaminophen, may be used to alleviate abdominal pain, discomfort, and fever associated with diverticulitis. NSAIDs should be used cautiously in individuals with diverticulitis, as they may exacerbate colonic inflammation, increase the risk of bleeding, or precipitate perforation. Acetaminophen is preferred for pain relief in diverticulitis, as it has minimal gastrointestinal side effects and does not interfere with colonic healing.

Antispasmodics: Antispasmodic agents, such as hyoscyamine, dicyclomine, or peppermint oil, may be used to relieve smooth muscle spasms, cramping, and abdominal discomfort associated with diverticulitis. These agents act locally on colonic smooth muscle to reduce hypermotility, spasm frequency, and visceral hypersensitivity. Antispasmodics are particularly useful in individuals with symptomatic diverticulosis or irritable bowel syndrome (IBS) features.

Probiotics: Probiotic supplements, containing beneficial bacteria strains (e.g., Lactobacillus, Bifidobacterium), may be used as adjunctive therapy in diverticulitis to restore colonic microbiota balance, enhance immune function, and reduce inflammation. Probiotics exert anti-inflammatory effects, improve epithelial barrier function, and inhibit pathogenic bacteria colonization within the gut. However, evidence supporting the use of probiotics in diverticulitis is limited, and further research is needed to elucidate their role in disease management.

Corticosteroids: Corticosteroids, such as prednisone or budesonide, may be used in select cases of severe or refractory diverticulitis to suppress inflammation, reduce edema, and alleviate symptoms. Corticosteroids have potent anti-inflammatory effects and may be beneficial in individuals with systemic manifestations, extensive colonic involvement, or corticosteroid-responsive disease. However, their long-term use is associated with significant adverse effects, including immunosuppression, osteoporosis, and metabolic complications, necessitating careful risk-benefit assessment.

Conclusion

In conclusion, conservative management plays a fundamental role in the comprehensive management of diverticulitis, encompassing dietary modifications and pharmacotherapy to alleviate symptoms, promote healing, and prevent disease recurrence. Dietary modifications, such as high-fiber diet, low-FODMAP diet, clear liquid diet, and low-residue diet, help optimize bowel function, minimize inflammation, and reduce symptomatic burden. Pharmacotherapy, including antibiotics, analgesics, antispasmodics, probiotics, and corticosteroids, targets inflammation, pain, infection, and symptomatic relief, offering adjunctive therapeutic options in diverticulitis management. However, individualized treatment plans should consider disease severity, clinical presentation, comorbidities, and patient preferences to optimize therapeutic outcomes and enhance quality of life. Further research into the efficacy, safety, and long-term effects of conservative management strategies in diverticulitis is warranted to refine treatment algorithms and improve patient care.

6.2 Surgical Management: Addressing Indications and Exploring Surgical Options in Diverticulitis

Surgical intervention plays a crucial role in the management of diverticulitis, particularly in cases of complications, recurrent disease, or refractory symptoms. This section provides an in-depth analysis of surgical management in diverticulitis, focusing on indications for surgery and the spectrum of surgical options available to patients.

Surgical Management

Surgical management of diverticulitis encompasses a range of procedures aimed at addressing complications, restoring colonic function, and preventing disease recurrence. While conservative measures remain the cornerstone of initial treatment, surgical intervention may be necessary in select cases to optimize patient outcomes and improve quality of life.

Indications for Surgery

The decision to proceed with surgical intervention in diverticulitis is guided by a combination of clinical, radiological, and endoscopic findings, with the primary goals of resolving complications, preventing disease progression, and improving long-term outcomes. Indications for surgery in diverticulitis include:

Complicated Diverticulitis: Complicated diverticulitis encompasses a spectrum of disease manifestations, including abscess formation, fistula formation, perforation, peritonitis, bowel obstruction, and recurrent episodes of acute inflammation. Surgical intervention is indicated in cases of complicated diverticulitis that fail to respond to conservative management, pose a significant risk of morbidity or mortality, or result in persistent symptoms and functional impairment.

Recurrent Disease: Recurrent episodes of diverticulitis, characterized by multiple acute exacerbations, frequent hospitalizations, or refractory symptoms despite medical therapy, may warrant consideration for surgical intervention. Recurrent disease is associated with an increased risk of complications, disease progression, and diminished quality of life, necessitating a proactive approach to disease management.

Failure of Conservative Management: Failure of

conservative management, including dietary modifications, pharmacotherapy, and lifestyle interventions, to adequately control symptoms, prevent disease recurrence, or improve colonic health may prompt consideration for surgical intervention. Persistent symptoms, functional impairment, and quality-of-life limitations despite optimal medical therapy indicate the need for a more definitive treatment approach.

Complications of Disease: Complications of diverticulitis, such as abscess formation, fistula formation, bowel obstruction, or perforation, may require surgical intervention to address acute pathology, alleviate symptoms, and prevent disease progression. Complications often arise from underlying inflammation, infection, or structural abnormalities within the colon and adjacent structures, necessitating prompt recognition and timely intervention.

Uncontrolled Symptoms: Uncontrolled symptoms of diverticulitis, including chronic abdominal pain, bloating, altered bowel habits, and quality-of-life limitations, may prompt consideration for surgical intervention in select cases. Persistent symptoms despite conservative management, pharmacotherapy, and lifestyle modifications may indicate underlying structural abnormalities, functional impairment, or refractory disease requiring surgical evaluation.

Surgical Options

Surgical management of diverticulitis encompasses a range of procedures tailored to individual patient characteristics, disease severity, and underlying pathology. Surgical options include:

Primary Resection and Anastomosis: Primary resection and anastomosis involve surgical resection of the affected colonic segment containing diverticula, followed by restoration of bowel continuity through an end-to-end or side-to-side anastomosis. This procedure is typically performed for uncomplicated diverticulitis without significant colonic involvement, strictures, or extensive disease burden. Primary resection and anastomosis aim to remove diseased tissue, alleviate symptoms, and prevent disease recurrence while preserving colonic function and continuity.

Hartmann's Procedure: Hartmann's procedure involves surgical resection of the affected colonic segment containing diverticula, closure of the rectal stump, and creation of an end colostomy to divert fecal flow away from the distal colon. This procedure is indicated for complicated diverticulitis with perforation, abscess formation, peritonitis, or significant colonic involvement unsuitable for primary anastomosis. Hartmann's procedure provides definitive treatment for acute complications of diverticulitis while avoiding the risks associated with immediate restoration of bowel continuity.

Colostomy or Ileostomy: Colostomy or ileostomy may be performed as temporary or permanent diversion procedures in cases of extensive colonic involvement, severe inflammation, or high risk of anastomotic complications. These procedures involve the creation of a stoma on the abdominal wall, through which fecal material is diverted into an external collection bag, bypassing the affected segment of the colon. Colostomy or ileostomy may be performed in conjunction with primary resection, Hartmann's procedure, or as a staged procedure in select cases of severe or refractory diverticulitis.

Laparoscopic or Robotic-Assisted Surgery: Laparoscopic or robotic-assisted surgery has emerged as a minimally invasive approach to diverticulitis management, offering advantages such as smaller incisions, reduced postoperative pain, faster recovery, and shorter hospital stays compared to traditional open surgery. These techniques allow for precise dissection, visualization, and tissue manipulation, facilitating colonic resection, anastomosis, and stoma creation with improved cosmesis and patient satisfaction. Laparoscopic or robotic-assisted surgery may be performed for both elective and emergent indications of diverticulitis, depending on patient factors and disease characteristics.

Surgical Complications and Considerations: Surgical management of diverticulitis is associated with potential complications, including anastomotic leakage, wound infection, hemorrhage, bowel obstruction, and stoma-related complications. Preoperative optimization, perioperative care, and postoperative monitoring are essential to minimize surgical risks, optimize outcomes, and facilitate patient recovery. Patient education, shared decision-making, and multidisciplinary collaboration are integral to ensuring informed consent, realistic expectations, and comprehensive care throughout the surgical journey.

Conclusion

In conclusion, surgical management plays a critical role in the comprehensive management of diverticulitis, addressing indications for surgery and exploring a spectrum of surgical options tailored to individual patient characteristics and disease severity. Indications for surgery in diverticulitis include complicated disease, recurrent episodes, failure of conservative management, complications of disease, and uncontrolled symptoms. Surgical options range from primary resection and anastomosis to Hartmann's procedure, colostomy or ileostomy, and laparoscopic or robotic-assisted surgery, depending on disease characteristics, patient factors, and surgical expertise. Surgical intervention aims to resolve acute complications, prevent disease recurrence, and improve long-term outcomes while minimizing surgical risks and optimizing patient recovery. Further research into the efficacy, safety, and long-term outcomes of surgical management strategies in diverticulitis is warranted to refine treatment algorithms and enhance patient care.

CHAPTER 7: PREVENTION AND LIFESTYLE MODIFICATIONS

7.1 Dietary Recommendations for Diverticulosis Management

Dietary recommendations play a crucial role in the management of diverticulosis, aiming to alleviate symptoms, prevent complications, and promote colonic health. This section provides comprehensive guidance on dietary recommendations for individuals with diverticulosis, focusing on fiber intake and fluid intake as key components of a healthy diet.

Dietary Recommendations

Dietary recommendations for diverticulosis management are centered around promoting bowel regularity, minimizing colonic irritation, and preventing diverticulitis exacerbations. Key dietary components include adequate fiber intake, sufficient fluid intake, and moderation of certain foods that may exacerbate symptoms or trigger diverticulitis flares.

Fiber Intake

Fiber intake is a cornerstone of dietary management in diverticulosis, as it plays a crucial role in maintaining bowel regularity, promoting stool bulk, and preventing constipation. Adequate fiber intake helps soften stool consistency, facilitate smooth bowel transit, and reduce the risk of fecal impaction within diverticula. Dietary fiber is classified into two main categories: soluble fiber and insoluble fiber.

Soluble Fiber: Soluble fiber, found in foods such as oats, barley, legumes, fruits, and vegetables, dissolves in water to form a gel-like substance in the digestive tract. Soluble fiber promotes stool softening, slows gastric emptying, and enhances nutrient absorption, leading to improved bowel regularity and reduced symptoms of constipation. Individuals with diverticulosis are encouraged to include soluble fiber-rich foods in their diet to support colonic health and prevent diverticulitis exacerbations.

Insoluble Fiber: Insoluble fiber, found in foods such as whole grains, wheat bran, nuts, seeds, and roughage, adds bulk to stool and promotes peristalsis in the digestive tract. Insoluble fiber acts as a natural laxative, speeding up bowel transit time and reducing the risk of fecal stagnation within diverticula. While insoluble fiber may exacerbate symptoms in some individuals with diverticulosis, it is generally well-tolerated and contributes to overall gastrointestinal health.

Recommended Fiber Intake: The recommended daily fiber intake for individuals with diverticulosis varies depending on age, sex, and dietary preferences. Generally, adults should aim for 25-30 grams of fiber per day, with an emphasis on consuming a diverse range of fiber-rich foods from both soluble and insoluble sources. Gradual introduction of fiber-rich foods into the diet, along with adequate fluid intake, can help minimize gastrointestinal discomfort and optimize bowel function.

Dietary Sources of Fiber: Dietary sources of fiber include fruits, vegetables, whole grains, legumes, nuts, seeds, and fiber supplements. Incorporating a variety of fiber-rich foods into meals and snacks ensures a balanced intake of soluble and insoluble fiber, supporting gastrointestinal health and preventing diverticulitis exacerbations. Examples of high-fiber foods include apples, pears, berries, broccoli, carrots, whole wheat bread, brown rice, lentils, beans, almonds, and chia seeds.

Fluid Intake

Fluid intake is essential for individuals with diverticulosis, as it helps maintain hydration, soften stool consistency, and facilitate smooth bowel transit. Adequate fluid intake is particularly important when increasing dietary fiber intake, as fiber absorbs water in the digestive tract and requires sufficient hydration to promote optimal bowel function.

Water: Water is the primary fluid source for maintaining hydration and supporting gastrointestinal health in individuals with diverticulosis. Drinking an adequate amount of water throughout the day helps prevent dehydration, soften stool consistency, and promote regular bowel movements. The recommended daily fluid intake varies depending on factors such as age, body weight, activity level, climate, and overall health status.

Fluid-Rich Foods: In addition to drinking water, individuals can increase their fluid intake by consuming fluid-rich foods such as fruits, vegetables, soups, and broths. Foods with high water content, such as watermelon, cucumber, celery, oranges, and lettuce, contribute to overall hydration and help meet daily fluid needs. Including a variety of fluid-rich foods in meals and snacks enhances hydration and supports gastrointestinal function.

Caffeine and Alcohol: While caffeine and alcohol-containing beverages such as coffee, tea, and alcoholic beverages can contribute to overall fluid intake, excessive consumption may have diuretic effects and lead to dehydration. Individuals with diverticulosis should limit caffeine and alcohol intake and balance them with non-caffeinated, non-alcoholic fluids to maintain hydration and prevent exacerbation of symptoms.

Hydration Strategies: To ensure adequate fluid intake, individuals with diverticulosis are encouraged to drink water regularly throughout the day, especially during meals and snacks, and to carry a reusable water bottle for convenient access to fluids. Monitoring urine color and frequency can serve as indicators of hydration status, with pale yellow urine signifying adequate hydration and dark yellow urine indicating potential dehydration.

Conclusion

In conclusion, dietary recommendations play a crucial role in the management of diverticulosis, with a focus on fiber intake and fluid intake as key components of a healthy diet. Adequate fiber intake supports bowel regularity, prevents constipation, and reduces the risk of diverticulitis exacerbations, while sufficient fluid intake maintains hydration, softens stool consistency, and facilitates smooth bowel transit. Incorporating a variety of fiber-rich foods and fluid sources into meals and snacks, along with mindful hydration strategies, helps support gastrointestinal health and optimize outcomes for individuals with diverticulosis. Further research into the efficacy, safety, and long-term effects of dietary interventions in diverticulosis management is warranted to refine recommendations and enhance patient care.

7.2 Exercise and Physical Activity in Diverticulosis Management

Exercise and physical activity are integral components of a holistic approach to managing diverticulosis, contributing to overall health, gastrointestinal function, and disease prevention. This section explores the benefits of exercise and physical activity in diverticulosis management, along with practical recommendations for incorporating these lifestyle interventions into daily routines.

Exercise and Physical Activity

Exercise and physical activity play multifaceted roles in promoting gastrointestinal health, alleviating symptoms, and reducing the risk of diverticulosis complications. Regular exercise has been associated with numerous physiological benefits, including improved bowel motility, enhanced immune function, reduced inflammation, and maintenance of healthy body weight. Incorporating exercise into daily life not only supports colonic health but also contributes to overall well-being and quality of life.

Benefits of Exercise and Physical Activity

Improved Bowel Function: Regular exercise stimulates bowel motility and accelerates colonic transit time, leading to more efficient waste elimination and reduced risk of constipation. Physical activity enhances peristaltic activity in the colon, promoting regular bowel movements and preventing fecal stagnation within diverticula.

Reduced Inflammation: Exercise exerts anti-inflammatory

effects throughout the body, including the gastrointestinal tract, by modulating immune responses, reducing oxidative stress, and enhancing tissue repair mechanisms. Chronic inflammation is implicated in the pathogenesis of diverticulosis and diverticulitis, making exercise a valuable adjunctive therapy in disease management.

Weight Management: Physical activity plays a key role in weight management and obesity prevention, which are known risk factors for diverticulosis development and progression. Regular exercise helps maintain a healthy body weight, reduces visceral adiposity, and improves metabolic parameters, thereby mitigating the risk of diverticular complications and associated comorbidities.

Stress Reduction: Exercise has stress-reducing effects on the body, promoting relaxation, mental well-being, and psychosocial resilience. Stress and anxiety have been linked to gastrointestinal symptoms and exacerbations of diverticulosis, making stress management an important aspect of disease management. Engaging in regular physical activity can help alleviate stress, improve mood, and enhance coping mechanisms.

Cardiovascular Health: Exercise improves cardiovascular fitness, reduces blood pressure, lowers cholesterol levels, and enhances endothelial function, contributing to overall cardiovascular health. Cardiovascular disease is a common comorbidity in individuals with diverticulosis, highlighting the importance of exercise in reducing cardiovascular risk and improving long-term outcomes.

Recommendations for Exercise and Physical Activity

Type of Exercise: A variety of exercise modalities can benefit individuals with diverticulosis, including aerobic exercise, strength training, flexibility exercises, and mind-body practices. Aerobic activities such as walking, jogging, cycling, swimming, and dancing promote cardiovascular health and stimulate bowel motility. Strength training exercises, such as weightlifting, resistance band exercises, and bodyweight exercises, enhance muscle tone and support abdominal and pelvic floor function. Flexibility exercises, such as yoga and stretching, improve joint mobility and relieve muscle tension. Mind-body practices, such as tai chi and qigong, promote relaxation, mindfulness, and stress reduction.

Frequency and Duration: The American Heart Association recommends at least 150 minutes of moderate-intensity aerobic exercise or 75 minutes of vigorous-intensity aerobic exercise per week, along with muscle-strengthening activities on two or more days per week. Individuals with diverticulosis should aim to incorporate a combination of aerobic, strength training, and flexibility exercises into their weekly routine to achieve optimal health benefits. Exercise sessions should be spread throughout the week to allow for adequate recovery and adaptation.

Intensity Level: Exercise intensity can be adjusted based on individual fitness levels, preferences, and goals. Moderate-intensity exercise, characterized by noticeable increases in heart rate and breathing, but still allowing for conversation, is suitable for most individuals with diverticulosis. Vigorous-intensity exercise, characterized by significant increases in heart rate and breathing, making conversation difficult, may be appropriate for those seeking higher fitness challenges. Beginners should start with low-to-moderate intensity activities and gradually progress to higher intensity levels as fitness improves.

Duration of Sessions: Exercise sessions should be tailored to individual preferences, time constraints, and physical capabilities. Aim for at least 30 minutes of moderate-intensity aerobic exercise on most days of the week, or shorter bouts of exercise accumulated throughout the day to meet the recommended weekly total. Strength training sessions can range from 20 to 60 minutes, depending on the number of exercises, sets, and repetitions performed. Flexibility and mind-body practices can be incorporated into daily routines for shorter durations, such as 10 to 30 minutes per session.

Progression and Variety: Gradually increase exercise duration, intensity, and frequency over time to promote fitness gains and prevent plateaus. Incorporate a variety of exercise modalities, including aerobic, strength training, flexibility, and mind-body practices, to ensure a well-rounded fitness program and prevent monotony. Cross-training, or alternating between different types of exercise, can help prevent overuse injuries, promote muscle balance, and maintain motivation.

Conclusion

In conclusion, exercise and physical activity are essential components of a comprehensive approach to managing diverticulosis, offering numerous benefits for gastrointestinal health, overall well-being, and disease prevention. Regular exercise promotes bowel regularity, reduces inflammation, supports weight management, alleviates stress, and improves cardiovascular fitness, contributing to optimal outcomes for individuals with diverticulosis. Incorporating a variety of exercise modalities into daily life, including aerobic, strength training, flexibility, and mind-body practices, enhances physical fitness, mental resilience, and quality of life. By adopting a balanced approach to exercise and physical activity, individuals with diverticulosis can optimize gastrointestinal function, minimize symptoms, and promote long-term health and wellness.

7.3 Smoking Cessation: A Vital Component of Diverticulosis Management

Smoking cessation is a critical aspect of diverticulosis management, offering numerous benefits for gastrointestinal health, disease prevention, and overall well-being. This section explores the detrimental effects of smoking on diverticular disease, the benefits of smoking cessation, and practical strategies for quitting smoking.

Smoking Cessation and Diverticulosis

Smoking has been identified as a significant risk factor for the development and progression of diverticular disease, including diverticulosis and diverticulitis. Cigarette smoking exerts a multitude of harmful effects on the gastrointestinal tract, contributing to inflammation, oxidative stress, impaired blood flow, and structural changes within the colon. Individuals who smoke are at increased risk of developing diverticulosis, experiencing recurrent episodes of diverticulitis, and suffering from complications such as perforation, abscess formation, and fistula formation.

Benefits of Smoking Cessation

Quitting smoking offers numerous health benefits for individuals with diverticulosis, including:

1. **Reduced Risk of Diverticular Complications**: Smoking cessation reduces the risk of diverticular complications such as diverticulitis exacerbations, perforation, abscess formation, and fistula formation. By eliminating exposure to harmful toxins and

carcinogens found in tobacco smoke, individuals can mitigate the inflammatory response, promote tissue healing, and prevent disease progression.

2. **Improved Gastrointestinal Health**: Smoking cessation promotes gastrointestinal health by reducing inflammation, oxidative stress, and mucosal damage within the colon. Quitting smoking allows the gastrointestinal tract to heal and recover from the detrimental effects of tobacco smoke, leading to improved colonic function, enhanced blood flow, and reduced susceptibility to diverticular disease.

3. **Enhanced Immune Function**: Smoking cessation enhances immune function and host defense mechanisms, reducing the risk of infections and inflammatory responses in individuals with diverticulosis. By quitting smoking, individuals can bolster their immune system, improve mucosal integrity, and enhance the body's ability to combat microbial pathogens associated with diverticular complications.

4. **Cardiovascular Benefits**: Smoking cessation has profound cardiovascular benefits, including reduced risk of heart disease, stroke, peripheral artery disease, and venous thromboembolism. Individuals with diverticulosis often have comorbid cardiovascular risk factors, making smoking cessation an important component of comprehensive disease management and risk reduction.

5. **Improved Quality of Life**: Smoking cessation improves overall quality of life by reducing symptoms, improving physical fitness, and enhancing psychological well-being. Quitting smoking allows individuals to enjoy better health, increased energy levels, and a sense of accomplishment, leading to enhanced quality of life and longevity.

Strategies for Smoking Cessation

Quitting smoking is challenging but achievable with the right strategies and support systems in place. Some effective strategies for smoking cessation include:

1. **Set a Quit Date**: Choose a specific date to quit smoking and commit to it wholeheartedly. Having a clear quit date helps mentally prepare for the transition and creates a sense of accountability.
2. **Seek Support**: Enlist the support of friends, family members, healthcare providers, or support groups to help navigate the quitting process. Supportive relationships provide encouragement, motivation, and accountability during challenging times.
3. **Utilize Nicotine Replacement Therapy (NRT)**: Nicotine replacement therapy, including nicotine patches, gum, lozenges, inhalers, and nasal sprays, can help alleviate withdrawal symptoms and cravings associated with quitting smoking. NRT provides a safer alternative to tobacco smoke while gradually weaning off nicotine dependence.
4. **Consider Prescription Medications**: Prescription medications such as varenicline (Chantix) and bupropion (Zyban) can help reduce cravings and withdrawal symptoms, making it easier to quit smoking. These medications work by targeting nicotine receptors in the brain and altering neurotransmitter activity associated with addiction.
5. **Practice Stress Management**: Develop healthy coping mechanisms for managing stress and anxiety without resorting to smoking. Engage in relaxation techniques such as deep breathing, meditation, yoga, or mindfulness to promote emotional well-being and resilience.

6. **Stay Active**: Incorporate regular physical activity and exercise into daily life to distract from cravings, reduce stress, and promote overall health. Physical activity serves as a positive outlet for energy, enhances mood, and boosts self-esteem during the quitting process.
7. **Avoid Triggers**: Identify and avoid smoking triggers such as social situations, alcohol consumption, and environmental cues that may tempt you to smoke. Replace unhealthy habits with healthier alternatives and create a smoke-free environment to support your quitting journey.
8. **Celebrate Milestones**: Celebrate small victories and milestones along the way, such as one day, one week, or one month smoke-free. Reward yourself for progress made and acknowledge the positive changes in your health and lifestyle.

Conclusion

In conclusion, smoking cessation is a vital component of diverticulosis management, offering numerous benefits for gastrointestinal health, disease prevention, and overall well-being. Quitting smoking reduces the risk of diverticular complications, improves gastrointestinal function, enhances immune function, reduces cardiovascular risk, and enhances quality of life for individuals with diverticulosis. By implementing effective strategies for smoking cessation, seeking support, and making positive lifestyle changes, individuals can successfully quit smoking and enjoy the many health benefits of a smoke-free life.

7.4 Weight Management in Diverticulosis

Weight management plays a significant role in the management of diverticulosis, contributing to symptom control, disease prevention, and overall health optimization. This section explores the impact of weight on diverticular disease, the benefits of weight management, and practical strategies for achieving and maintaining a healthy weight.

Weight Management and Diverticulosis

Maintaining a healthy weight is important for individuals with diverticulosis, as obesity and excess adiposity are associated with an increased risk of disease development, progression, and complications. Excess body weight contributes to systemic inflammation, altered colonic motility, increased intraluminal pressure, and impaired immune function, all of which may exacerbate diverticular symptoms and predispose to diverticulitis flares.

Benefits of Weight Management

Effective weight management offers numerous benefits for individuals with diverticulosis, including:

1. **Reduced Risk of Diverticular Complications**: Weight management helps reduce the risk of diverticular complications such as diverticulitis exacerbations, perforation, abscess formation, and fistula formation. Achieving and maintaining a healthy weight lowers intraluminal pressure, promotes colonic health, and mitigates the inflammatory response associated with diverticular disease.
2. **Improved Gastrointestinal Function**: Maintaining a healthy weight supports optimal gastrointestinal function by reducing colonic inflammation, enhancing bowel motility, and promoting regular bowel movements. Weight management strategies

such as dietary modifications, physical activity, and lifestyle changes help alleviate symptoms of constipation, bloating, and abdominal discomfort commonly associated with diverticulosis.

3. **Enhanced Immune Function**: Weight management contributes to enhanced immune function and host defense mechanisms, reducing the risk of infections and inflammatory responses in individuals with diverticulosis. Achieving a healthy weight improves immune surveillance, enhances tissue repair, and strengthens mucosal integrity, thereby reducing susceptibility to diverticular complications.

4. **Cardiometabolic Benefits**: Weight management has cardiometabolic benefits, including improved lipid profiles, blood glucose control, and blood pressure regulation. Individuals with diverticulosis often have comorbidities such as hypertension, dyslipidemia, and metabolic syndrome, making weight management an essential component of comprehensive disease management and risk reduction.

5. **Enhanced Quality of Life**: Achieving and maintaining a healthy weight improves overall quality of life by reducing symptoms, improving physical function, and enhancing psychological well-being. Weight management empowers individuals to take control of their health, increase energy levels, and enjoy a higher quality of life free from the burden of excess weight.

Strategies for Weight Management

Effective weight management involves adopting a multifaceted approach that encompasses dietary modifications, physical activity, behavior change, and lifestyle interventions. Some practical strategies for weight management in individuals with diverticulosis include:

1. **Balanced Diet**: Follow a balanced diet rich in fruits, vegetables, whole grains, lean proteins, and healthy fats to promote satiety, regulate appetite, and support weight loss or weight maintenance. Emphasize fiber-rich foods, such as fruits, vegetables, legumes, and whole grains, which promote bowel regularity and aid in weight management.
2. **Portion Control**: Practice portion control and mindful eating to avoid overeating and promote weight loss or weight maintenance. Use smaller plates, bowls, and utensils to control portion sizes, and pay attention to hunger and fullness cues to prevent excessive calorie intake.
3. **Regular Physical Activity**: Engage in regular physical activity and exercise to promote calorie expenditure, improve fitness, and support weight management. Aim for at least 150 minutes of moderate-intensity aerobic exercise or 75 minutes of vigorous-intensity aerobic exercise per week, along with muscle-strengthening activities on two or more days per week.
4. **Behavioral Strategies**: Implement behavioral strategies such as goal setting, self-monitoring, stimulus control, and social support to facilitate adherence to weight management goals. Set realistic, achievable goals, track progress regularly, identify and address barriers to success, and enlist the support of friends, family members, or healthcare providers for encouragement and accountability.
5. **Lifestyle Modifications**: Make lifestyle modifications that promote overall health and well-being, including adequate sleep, stress management, hydration, and avoidance of excessive alcohol consumption. Prioritize self-care activities that support physical, mental, and emotional health, thereby facilitating sustainable weight management.

6. **Professional Support**: Seek professional support from registered dietitians, nutritionists, or healthcare providers with expertise in weight management to develop personalized nutrition plans, exercise prescriptions, and behavior change strategies. Collaborate with a multidisciplinary team to address underlying medical conditions, metabolic factors, and psychosocial determinants of weight management.

Conclusion

In conclusion, weight management is an essential component of diverticulosis management, offering numerous benefits for gastrointestinal health, disease prevention, and overall well-being. Effective weight management reduces the risk of diverticular complications, improves gastrointestinal function, enhances immune function, and enhances quality of life for individuals with diverticulosis. By adopting a balanced approach to diet, physical activity, behavior change, and lifestyle interventions, individuals can achieve and maintain a healthy weight, optimize gastrointestinal health, and reduce the burden of diverticular disease.

7.5 Stress Reduction Techniques for Diverticulosis Management

Stress reduction techniques play a vital role in the management of diverticulosis, as stress can exacerbate symptoms, trigger flares, and impact overall well-being. This section explores the relationship between stress and diverticular disease, the benefits of stress reduction techniques, and practical strategies for incorporating stress management into daily life.

Stress Reduction Techniques

Chronic stress has been implicated in the pathogenesis and exacerbation of diverticular disease, contributing to alterations in gastrointestinal motility, immune function, and inflammatory responses. Stress reduction techniques offer a holistic approach to diverticulosis management, promoting relaxation, emotional well-being, and improved coping mechanisms. By incorporating stress management strategies into daily life, individuals with diverticulosis can mitigate the impact of stress on their symptoms and overall health.

Benefits of Stress Reduction Techniques

Effective stress reduction techniques offer numerous benefits for individuals with diverticulosis, including:

1. **Symptom Control**: Stress reduction techniques help alleviate symptoms such as abdominal pain, bloating, and altered bowel habits associated with diverticulosis. By reducing stress levels, individuals can minimize gastrointestinal discomfort and improve quality of life.
2. **Disease Prevention**: Chronic stress has been linked to the development and progression of diverticular disease, making stress reduction an important aspect of disease prevention. By managing stress effectively, individuals can reduce the risk of diverticular complications and promote gastrointestinal health.
3. **Immune Modulation**: Stress reduction techniques modulate immune function, enhancing host defense mechanisms and reducing susceptibility to infections and inflammatory responses. By promoting immune resilience, stress management supports overall health and well-being in individuals with diverticulosis.
4. **Psychological Well-being**: Stress reduction techniques promote psychological well-being by

reducing anxiety, depression, and psychological distress associated with chronic illness. By fostering emotional resilience and coping skills, stress management enhances mental health outcomes and improves overall quality of life.

5. **Enhanced Coping Mechanisms**: Stress reduction techniques equip individuals with diverticulosis with effective coping mechanisms to navigate challenges and setbacks associated with their condition. By fostering adaptive coping strategies, stress management enhances resilience and promotes proactive self-care behaviors.

Practical Strategies for Stress Reduction

Effective stress reduction techniques encompass a variety of strategies that promote relaxation, mindfulness, and emotional well-being. Some practical techniques for managing stress in individuals with diverticulosis include:

1. **Deep Breathing Exercises**: Practice deep breathing exercises to promote relaxation, reduce muscle tension, and alleviate stress. Focus on slow, deep breaths, inhaling deeply through the nose and exhaling slowly through the mouth, to engage the parasympathetic nervous system and induce a state of calm.

2. **Mindfulness Meditation**: Incorporate mindfulness meditation into daily routines to cultivate present moment awareness, acceptance, and non-judgmental observation of thoughts and sensations. Engage in guided meditation practices, mindfulness-based stress reduction (MBSR) programs, or mindfulness apps to develop mindfulness skills and reduce stress levels.

3. **Progressive Muscle Relaxation (PMR)**: Practice progressive muscle relaxation techniques to

systematically tense and relax muscle groups throughout the body, promoting physical relaxation and stress relief. Start by tensing each muscle group for a few seconds, then release and relax, progressing from head to toe or vice versa.
4. **Yoga and Tai Chi**: Engage in yoga, tai chi, or qigong practices to promote relaxation, flexibility, and mind-body awareness. These mind-body practices combine physical postures, breathing techniques, and meditation to reduce stress, improve mobility, and enhance overall well-being.
5. **Nature Therapy**: Spend time in nature, such as walking in a park, hiking in the woods, or gardening, to promote relaxation, reduce stress, and improve mood. Nature therapy, or ecotherapy, has been shown to have beneficial effects on mental health and well-being, offering a natural antidote to urban stressors.
6. **Social Support**: Seek support from friends, family members, support groups, or mental health professionals to share concerns, express emotions, and receive encouragement during times of stress. Social support provides a sense of connection, belonging, and validation, buffering the impact of stress and promoting resilience.
7. **Healthy Lifestyle Habits**: Adopt healthy lifestyle habits such as regular physical activity, balanced nutrition, adequate sleep, and relaxation techniques to support overall well-being and stress management. Prioritize self-care activities that promote physical, mental, and emotional health, fostering resilience and enhancing coping mechanisms.

Conclusion

In conclusion, stress reduction techniques play a crucial role in the management of diverticulosis, offering numerous benefits for symptom control, disease prevention, and overall well-being. By incorporating stress management strategies into daily life, individuals with diverticulosis can mitigate the impact of stress on their symptoms and quality of life. Practical techniques such as deep breathing exercises, mindfulness meditation, progressive muscle relaxation, and mind-body practices promote relaxation, reduce tension, and enhance coping mechanisms. By prioritizing self-care, fostering social support, and adopting healthy lifestyle habits, individuals can effectively manage stress and optimize their health and well-being in the context of diverticular disease.

CHAPTER 8: HOLISTIC APPROACHES TO DIVERTICULOSIS MANAGEMENT

8.1 Role of Probiotics and Prebiotics in Diverticulosis Management

Probiotics and prebiotics play important roles in the management of diverticulosis by modulating the gut microbiota, promoting gastrointestinal health, and reducing the risk of diverticular complications. This section explores the mechanisms of action, potential benefits, and practical considerations regarding the use of probiotics and prebiotics in diverticulosis management.

Role of Probiotics

Probiotics are live microorganisms that confer health benefits when consumed in adequate amounts. They can help restore microbial balance in the gut, enhance immune function, and improve gastrointestinal symptoms associated with diverticulosis. Several mechanisms underlie the beneficial effects of probiotics in diverticular disease:

1. **Microbial Balance**: Probiotics help restore microbial balance in the gut by promoting the growth of beneficial bacteria and inhibiting the growth of pathogenic microbes. By modulating the composition and diversity of the gut microbiota, probiotics contribute to a healthier gut environment and reduced inflammation.
2. **Immune Modulation**: Probiotics interact with the gut-associated lymphoid tissue (GALT) and mucosal immune system, enhancing immune function and reducing inflammation. By stimulating the production of anti-inflammatory cytokines and suppressing pro-inflammatory mediators, probiotics help regulate immune responses and maintain gut homeostasis.
3. **Short-Chain Fatty Acid (SCFA) Production**: Probiotics ferment dietary fibers and prebiotics in the colon, leading to the production of short-chain fatty acids (SCFAs) such as butyrate, acetate, and propionate. SCFAs provide energy for colonocytes, support mucosal integrity, and exert anti-inflammatory effects, contributing to gastrointestinal health and symptom relief.
4. **Mucosal Protection**: Probiotics enhance mucosal barrier function and protect against epithelial damage by promoting the production of mucin, strengthening tight junctions, and inhibiting pathogen adhesion. By reinforcing the gut epithelium, probiotics help prevent bacterial translocation, mucosal injury, and inflammation.
5. **Symptom Relief**: Probiotics alleviate gastrointestinal symptoms such as bloating, gas, constipation, and diarrhea associated with diverticulosis. By modulating

gut motility, improving stool consistency, and reducing fermentation of undigested carbohydrates, probiotics help alleviate symptoms and improve overall quality of life.

Practical Considerations for Probiotic Use

When considering probiotic supplementation for diverticulosis management, several practical considerations should be taken into account:

1. **Strain Selection**: Choose probiotic strains with proven efficacy and safety in the management of gastrointestinal disorders, including Lactobacillus and Bifidobacterium species. Look for strains with documented health benefits, such as Lactobacillus rhamnosus GG, Lactobacillus acidophilus, Bifidobacterium lactis, and Bifidobacterium longum.
2. **Dosage**: Follow recommended dosage guidelines provided by the manufacturer or healthcare provider. Probiotic dosages may vary depending on the strain, formulation, and intended use. Start with a lower dosage and gradually increase as needed, monitoring for any adverse effects or gastrointestinal symptoms.
3. **Formulation**: Choose probiotic formulations that ensure viability and stability of the live microorganisms throughout storage and transit. Look for products with guaranteed potency, enteric-coated capsules, or refrigerated formulations to optimize survival of probiotic bacteria until consumption.
4. **Combination Therapies**: Consider combining probiotics with prebiotics, dietary fibers, or synbiotics (combination of probiotics and prebiotics) to enhance their efficacy and synergistic effects. Prebiotics serve as substrates for probiotic growth and fermentation, enhancing their survival and activity in the gut.

5. **Duration of Use**: Use probiotics consistently and for an appropriate duration to achieve desired therapeutic effects. Long-term supplementation may be necessary to maintain microbial balance and prevent recurrence of symptoms in individuals with diverticulosis.

Role of Prebiotics

Prebiotics are non-digestible dietary fibers that selectively stimulate the growth and activity of beneficial bacteria in the gut, such as Bifidobacteria and Lactobacilli. By serving as substrates for probiotic fermentation, prebiotics promote the proliferation of beneficial bacteria, enhance microbial diversity, and improve gastrointestinal health. Several mechanisms underlie the beneficial effects of prebiotics in diverticular disease:

1. **Selective Stimulation**: Prebiotics selectively stimulate the growth and activity of beneficial bacteria in the gut, such as Bifidobacteria and Lactobacilli, while inhibiting the growth of pathogenic microbes. By promoting a healthier gut microbiota composition, prebiotics support gastrointestinal health and reduce the risk of diverticular complications.
2. **Fermentation and SCFA Production**: Prebiotics are fermented by probiotic bacteria in the colon, leading to the production of short-chain fatty acids (SCFAs) such as butyrate, acetate, and propionate. SCFAs provide energy for colonocytes, regulate immune function, and exert anti-inflammatory effects, contributing to gut health and symptom relief.
3. **Improved Bowel Function**: Prebiotics promote bowel regularity, soften stool consistency, and alleviate symptoms of constipation associated with diverticulosis. By increasing fecal bulk and water content, prebiotics facilitate smooth bowel transit and

reduce the risk of fecal impaction within diverticula.
4. **Mucosal Protection**: Prebiotics enhance mucosal barrier function and protect against epithelial damage by stimulating the production of mucin, strengthening tight junctions, and enhancing mucosal immunity. By fortifying the gut epithelium, prebiotics help prevent bacterial translocation, mucosal injury, and inflammation.
5. **Symptom Relief**: Prebiotics alleviate gastrointestinal symptoms such as bloating, gas, and abdominal discomfort in individuals with diverticulosis. By modulating gut motility, promoting microbial balance, and enhancing SCFA production, prebiotics improve overall gut function and symptom control.

Practical Considerations for Prebiotic Use

When incorporating prebiotics into the diet for diverticulosis management, several practical considerations should be taken into account:

1. **Dietary Sources**: Include prebiotic-rich foods in the diet, such as fruits, vegetables, whole grains, legumes, nuts, and seeds. Choose a variety of prebiotic-containing foods to ensure a diverse intake of dietary fibers and promote microbial diversity in the gut.
2. **Fiber Content**: Pay attention to the fiber content of foods and aim to meet recommended daily fiber intake goals. Gradually increase fiber intake to minimize gastrointestinal discomfort and allow for adaptation of the gut microbiota to dietary changes.
3. **Hydration**: Drink plenty of fluids when increasing fiber intake to prevent constipation and promote optimal bowel function. Adequate hydration is essential for softening stool consistency, facilitating smooth bowel transit, and supporting the

fermentation of prebiotic fibers by gut bacteria.
4. **Supplementation**: Consider prebiotic supplements or functional foods fortified with prebiotic fibers if dietary intake is inadequate or if additional support is needed. Choose supplements that contain well-tolerated prebiotic fibers such as inulin, oligofructose, galactooligosaccharides (GOS), or resistant starch.
5. **Individual Tolerance**: Monitor individual tolerance to prebiotic-rich foods and supplements, as some individuals may experience gastrointestinal symptoms such as bloating, gas, or diarrhea with increased fiber intake. Start with small amounts and gradually increase as tolerated to minimize discomfort.

Conclusion

In conclusion, probiotics and prebiotics play important roles in the management of diverticulosis by modulating the gut microbiota, promoting gastrointestinal health, and reducing the risk of diverticular complications. Probiotics help restore microbial balance, enhance immune function, and alleviate gastrointestinal symptoms, while prebiotics selectively stimulate the growth of beneficial bacteria, improve bowel function, and support mucosal protection. By incorporating probiotics and prebiotics into the diet or as supplements, individuals with diverticulosis can optimize gut health, alleviate symptoms, and promote overall well-being. However, it's essential to choose appropriate probiotic strains, formulations, and prebiotic sources, and to monitor individual tolerance to dietary changes to maximize benefits and minimize adverse effects.

8.2 Herbal Remedies and Supplements in Diverticulosis Management

Herbal remedies and supplements are often explored as complementary or alternative treatments for diverticulosis, offering potential benefits for symptom relief, gut health, and overall well-being. This section examines the role of herbal remedies and supplements in diverticulosis management, their mechanisms of action, and practical considerations for their use.

Herbal Remedies

Herbal remedies have been used for centuries in traditional medicine systems to alleviate gastrointestinal symptoms, promote gut health, and support overall wellness. While scientific evidence supporting the efficacy of herbal remedies in diverticulosis is limited, some herbs may offer potential benefits through their anti-inflammatory, antimicrobial, and digestive properties. Here are a few herbal remedies that have been studied or traditionally used for diverticulosis management:

1. **Psyllium Husk**: Psyllium husk, derived from the Plantago ovata plant, is a soluble fiber supplement commonly used to alleviate constipation and promote bowel regularity. Psyllium husk absorbs water in the colon, forming a gel-like substance that softens stool consistency and facilitates smooth bowel transit. By increasing fecal bulk and promoting regular bowel movements, psyllium husk may help alleviate symptoms of constipation associated with diverticulosis.

2. **Peppermint Oil**: Peppermint oil is well-known for its antispasmodic and carminative properties, making it a popular remedy for digestive issues such as bloating, gas, and abdominal discomfort. Peppermint oil relaxes smooth muscle in the gastrointestinal tract, reducing spasms and discomfort associated with diverticulosis. While limited research exists on the use of peppermint oil specifically for diverticulosis, it may offer symptomatic relief for some individuals.
3. **Marshmallow Root**: Marshmallow root contains mucilage, a gel-like substance that coats and soothes the gastrointestinal tract, providing relief from inflammation and irritation. Marshmallow root has been traditionally used to alleviate symptoms of gastrointestinal conditions such as gastritis, ulcers, and irritable bowel syndrome (IBS). While research on marshmallow root for diverticulosis is lacking, its demulcent properties may offer potential benefits for soothing inflamed mucosa and alleviating symptoms.
4. **Slippery Elm Bark**: Slippery elm bark contains mucilage and other compounds that coat the digestive tract, providing a protective barrier and promoting healing of inflamed tissues. Slippery elm bark has been used traditionally to alleviate symptoms of gastrointestinal conditions such as gastritis, ulcers, and inflammatory bowel disease (IBD). While evidence specific to diverticulosis is limited, slippery elm bark may offer symptomatic relief for individuals experiencing abdominal discomfort and inflammation.

Dietary Supplements

Dietary supplements, including vitamins, minerals, and other nutrients, are commonly used to support overall health and well-being. While dietary supplements are not a substitute for a healthy diet and lifestyle, they may offer additional support for individuals with diverticulosis by addressing nutrient deficiencies, promoting gut health, and supporting immune function. Here are some dietary supplements that may be relevant to diverticulosis management:

1. **Fiber Supplements**: Fiber supplements such as psyllium husk, methylcellulose, and wheat dextrin can help increase dietary fiber intake and alleviate symptoms of constipation associated with diverticulosis. Fiber supplements should be used with caution and adequate hydration to prevent gastrointestinal discomfort and obstruction.
2. **Probiotics**: Probiotic supplements contain live beneficial bacteria that may help restore microbial balance in the gut, support immune function, and alleviate gastrointestinal symptoms. While evidence supporting the use of probiotics for diverticulosis is limited, certain strains such as Lactobacillus and Bifidobacterium species may offer potential benefits for gut health.
3. **Digestive Enzymes**: Digestive enzyme supplements contain enzymes such as amylase, lipase, and protease that help break down carbohydrates, fats, and proteins in the digestive tract. Digestive enzyme supplements may support digestion and nutrient absorption in individuals with diverticulosis who experience digestive issues such as bloating, gas, and abdominal discomfort.
4. **Omega-3 Fatty Acids**: Omega-3 fatty acid supplements, such as fish oil or flaxseed oil, contain essential fatty acids with anti-inflammatory properties that may help reduce inflammation and promote cardiovascular health. While evidence specific to diverticulosis is limited, omega-3 fatty

acids may offer potential benefits for reducing inflammation and supporting overall well-being.

Practical Considerations for Herbal Remedies and Supplements

When considering the use of herbal remedies and supplements for diverticulosis management, it's important to approach with caution and consult with a healthcare provider, particularly if you have underlying medical conditions or are taking medications. Here are some practical considerations to keep in mind:

1. **Consultation with Healthcare Provider**: Before starting any herbal remedies or supplements, consult with a healthcare provider to discuss potential benefits, risks, and interactions with medications or existing health conditions. Some herbal remedies and supplements may interact with medications or exacerbate underlying health issues.
2. **Quality and Safety**: Choose high-quality herbal remedies and supplements from reputable manufacturers that adhere to good manufacturing practices (GMP) and undergo third-party testing for purity, potency, and safety. Look for standardized extracts and certified organic products when available.
3. **Dosage and Administration**: Follow recommended dosage guidelines provided by the manufacturer or healthcare provider. Start with a lower dosage and gradually increase as needed, monitoring for any adverse effects or gastrointestinal symptoms. Some herbal remedies and supplements may require time to exert their effects, so be patient and consistent with usage.
4. **Potential Side Effects**: Be aware of potential side effects or adverse reactions associated with herbal

remedies and supplements. Common side effects may include gastrointestinal upset, allergic reactions, or interactions with medications. Discontinue use and consult with a healthcare provider if you experience any adverse effects.
5. **Monitoring and Evaluation**: Regularly monitor your response to herbal remedies and supplements and evaluate their effectiveness in alleviating symptoms and improving overall well-being. Keep track of any changes in symptoms, medication interactions, or adverse effects, and communicate with your healthcare provider as needed.

Conclusion

In conclusion, herbal remedies and supplements may offer potential benefits for individuals with diverticulosis by addressing symptoms, promoting gut health, and supporting overall well-being. While scientific evidence supporting their efficacy in diverticular disease is limited, certain herbs and dietary supplements may have anti-inflammatory, digestive, and immunomodulatory properties that could be beneficial. However, it's essential to approach the use of herbal remedies and supplements with caution, consult with a healthcare provider, and prioritize quality, safety, and appropriate dosage. Integrating herbal remedies and supplements into a comprehensive treatment plan alongside dietary and lifestyle modifications may help individuals with diverticulosis optimize their health and manage their condition effectively.

8.3 Mind-Body Practices in Diverticulosis Management

Mind-body practices encompass a range of techniques and

therapies that promote the integration of the mind and body to enhance health, well-being, and self-awareness. These practices have gained recognition for their potential benefits in managing various health conditions, including gastrointestinal disorders like diverticulosis. This section explores the role of specific mind-body practices, including meditation, yoga, and acupuncture, in diverticulosis management.

Meditation

Meditation is a mindfulness practice that involves focusing attention, cultivating awareness, and promoting relaxation to achieve a state of mental clarity and emotional balance. Meditation techniques vary but commonly include focused attention on breath, visualization, mantra repetition, or body scanning. Meditation offers several potential benefits for individuals with diverticulosis:

- **Stress Reduction**: Meditation promotes relaxation and reduces the physiological and psychological effects of stress, including elevated cortisol levels, sympathetic nervous system activation, and emotional reactivity. By inducing a state of calm and equanimity, meditation helps mitigate the impact of stress on gastrointestinal symptoms and overall well-being.
- **Pain Management**: Meditation can help individuals cope with chronic pain, including abdominal discomfort associated with diverticulosis. By cultivating non-judgmental awareness of pain sensations and developing acceptance and resilience, meditation fosters a sense of control and reduces pain perception.
- **Gut-Brain Connection**: Meditation influences the gut-brain axis, a bidirectional communication network linking the central nervous system (CNS) and the enteric nervous system (ENS). By modulating

neurotransmitter activity, neuroendocrine responses, and autonomic nervous system function, meditation influences gastrointestinal function, immune responses, and gut microbiota composition.

- **Emotional Well-being**: Meditation enhances emotional regulation, self-awareness, and compassion, fostering psychological well-being and resilience in individuals with diverticulosis. By cultivating present moment awareness and non-reactive acceptance of thoughts and emotions, meditation promotes adaptive coping mechanisms and reduces psychological distress.

Yoga

Yoga is a mind-body practice that integrates physical postures (asanas), breath control (pranayama), and meditation to promote holistic health and well-being. Yoga offers numerous potential benefits for individuals with diverticulosis, including:

- **Gastrointestinal Health**: Certain yoga poses and practices can stimulate digestion, improve bowel motility, and alleviate symptoms of constipation or bloating associated with diverticulosis. Poses that involve twisting, forward bending, and gentle compression of the abdomen may promote peristalsis and relieve gastrointestinal discomfort.
- **Stress Reduction**: Yoga incorporates breath awareness, relaxation techniques, and mindfulness practices that promote stress reduction and relaxation. By synchronizing breath with movement and cultivating mindfulness of bodily sensations, yoga induces a state of calm and tranquility, reducing stress-related exacerbations of diverticular symptoms.
- **Physical Fitness**: Regular practice of yoga enhances flexibility, strength, and cardiovascular

fitness, supporting overall physical health and well-being. Engaging in gentle yoga sequences or restorative practices can improve mobility, posture, and functional movement patterns, reducing musculoskeletal tension and discomfort.
- **Mind-Body Awareness**: Yoga cultivates mind-body awareness, promoting conscious alignment, proprioception, and body-mind connection. By fostering introspection, self-compassion, and acceptance of bodily sensations, yoga helps individuals develop a deeper understanding of their physical and emotional needs, facilitating self-care and symptom management.

Acupuncture

Acupuncture is a traditional Chinese medicine (TCM) therapy that involves the insertion of thin needles into specific points on the body to stimulate energy flow (Qi) and restore balance to the body's systems. While scientific evidence supporting acupuncture for diverticulosis is limited, some individuals may experience symptom relief and improved well-being with acupuncture treatment. Potential benefits of acupuncture for diverticulosis management include:

- **Pain Relief**: Acupuncture can help alleviate abdominal pain, cramping, and discomfort associated with diverticulosis by modulating pain perception and reducing inflammation. Acupuncture stimulates the release of endorphins and neurotransmitters that inhibit pain signals and promote relaxation.
- **Stress Reduction**: Acupuncture promotes relaxation, reduces sympathetic nervous system activity, and modulates stress hormone levels, contributing to overall stress reduction and emotional well-being. By balancing the autonomic nervous system and

promoting parasympathetic dominance, acupuncture helps mitigate the effects of stress on gastrointestinal function.

- **Regulation of Gastrointestinal Function**: Acupuncture may influence gastrointestinal motility, secretion, and visceral sensitivity through its effects on neural pathways, neurotransmitter release, and endocrine signaling. By regulating peristalsis, sphincter tone, and gut-brain communication, acupuncture supports optimal gastrointestinal function and symptom control.
- **Immune Modulation**: Acupuncture has immunomodulatory effects, including regulation of inflammatory cytokines, enhancement of immune cell activity, and modulation of immune responses. By modulating immune function and reducing systemic inflammation, acupuncture may support immune resilience and reduce the risk of diverticular complications.

Practical Considerations for Mind-Body Practices

When incorporating mind-body practices such as meditation, yoga, and acupuncture into diverticulosis management, it's important to consider the following practical considerations:

- **Individualized Approach**: Mind-body practices should be tailored to individual preferences, needs, and capabilities. Choose practices that resonate with you and that you enjoy, whether it's meditation, yoga, acupuncture, or a combination of modalities.
- **Safety and Accessibility**: Practice mind-body techniques safely and mindfully, respecting your body's limitations and avoiding excessive strain or discomfort. Seek guidance from qualified instructors or healthcare providers, particularly if you have

underlying health conditions or physical limitations.
- **Consistency and Persistence**: Consistent practice is key to reaping the benefits of mind-body techniques. Set aside dedicated time for practice, integrate techniques into daily routines, and approach with patience and persistence. Progress may be gradual, so be open to the process and observe changes over time.
- **Integration with Conventional Care**: Mind-body practices should complement, not replace, conventional medical care for diverticulosis. Inform your healthcare provider about your use of mind-body techniques, and incorporate them into a comprehensive treatment plan alongside dietary modifications, medication management, and other therapies.

Conclusion

In conclusion, mind-body practices such as meditation, yoga, and acupuncture offer valuable tools for individuals with diverticulosis to manage symptoms, promote gut health, and enhance overall well-being. These practices harness the interconnectedness of the mind and body to reduce stress, alleviate pain, improve gastrointestinal function, and support emotional resilience. By integrating mind-body techniques into daily life alongside conventional medical care, individuals with diverticulosis can optimize their health, enhance symptom management, and cultivate a greater sense of well-being.

8.4 Integrative Medicine Approaches in Diverticulosis Management

Integrative medicine approaches combine conventional medical treatments with complementary and alternative therapies to address the physical, emotional, and spiritual aspects of health and wellness. By integrating evidence-based practices from both conventional and holistic medicine, integrative approaches offer a comprehensive and personalized approach to diverticulosis management. This section explores various integrative medicine approaches that may benefit individuals with diverticulosis, including dietary interventions, lifestyle modifications, supplements, mind-body practices, and other holistic therapies.

Dietary Interventions

Dietary interventions play a central role in integrative medicine approaches to diverticulosis management, aiming to optimize gut health, alleviate symptoms, and prevent diverticular complications. Key dietary strategies include:

- **High-Fiber Diet**: Emphasize a high-fiber diet rich in fruits, vegetables, whole grains, legumes, and nuts to promote bowel regularity, soften stool consistency, and reduce the risk of constipation and diverticular complications. Adequate dietary fiber intake helps maintain optimal gut motility and prevents fecal impaction within diverticula.
- **Hydration**: Stay well-hydrated by drinking plenty of fluids, particularly water, to soften stool consistency, facilitate smooth bowel transit, and prevent dehydration. Adequate hydration is essential for optimizing gastrointestinal function and supporting the fermentation of dietary fibers by gut bacteria.
- **Low-FODMAP Diet**: Consider a low-FODMAP (fermentable oligosaccharides, disaccharides, monosaccharides, and polyols) diet for individuals with diverticulosis who experience symptoms

of bloating, gas, and abdominal discomfort. This temporary elimination diet restricts certain fermentable carbohydrates that may exacerbate gastrointestinal symptoms, allowing for symptom relief and identification of trigger foods.
- **Probiotics and Prebiotics**: Incorporate probiotic-rich foods (e.g., yogurt, kefir, fermented vegetables) and prebiotic-containing foods (e.g., garlic, onions, leeks, asparagus, bananas) into the diet to promote a healthy gut microbiota, enhance immune function, and support gastrointestinal health. Probiotic and prebiotic supplements may also be beneficial for some individuals.

Lifestyle Modifications

Lifestyle modifications are integral components of integrative medicine approaches to diverticulosis management, focusing on optimizing overall health and well-being. Key lifestyle strategies include:

- **Regular Physical Activity**: Engage in regular physical activity, such as walking, swimming, cycling, or yoga, to promote gastrointestinal motility, reduce stress, and maintain overall fitness. Aim for at least 30 minutes of moderate-intensity exercise most days of the week, or as recommended by a healthcare provider.
- **Stress Management**: Practice stress reduction techniques such as meditation, yoga, deep breathing exercises, or mindfulness practices to reduce stress levels, promote relaxation, and alleviate symptoms of diverticulosis. Stress management techniques help mitigate the impact of psychological stress on gastrointestinal function and overall well-being.
- **Smoking Cessation**: Quit smoking if you are a smoker, as smoking has been associated with an increased

risk of diverticular complications and may exacerbate symptoms of diverticulosis. Seek support from healthcare providers, smoking cessation programs, or support groups to successfully quit smoking and improve gastrointestinal health.
- **Healthy Sleep Habits**: Prioritize adequate sleep and establish healthy sleep habits to support overall health and well-being. Aim for 7-9 hours of quality sleep per night, maintain a consistent sleep schedule, create a relaxing bedtime routine, and optimize sleep environment for restorative sleep.

Herbal Remedies and Supplements

Herbal remedies and supplements may complement conventional medical treatments in integrative medicine approaches to diverticulosis management. Key herbal remedies and supplements that may be beneficial include:

- **Psyllium Husk**: Psyllium husk, a soluble fiber supplement, can help increase dietary fiber intake, promote bowel regularity, and alleviate symptoms of constipation associated with diverticulosis.
- **Probiotics and Prebiotics**: Probiotic supplements containing beneficial bacteria (e.g., Lactobacillus, Bifidobacterium) and prebiotic fibers can help restore microbial balance in the gut, support immune function, and improve gastrointestinal health.
- **Peppermint Oil**: Peppermint oil supplements may offer symptomatic relief for abdominal discomfort, bloating, and gas associated with diverticulosis, due to their antispasmodic and carminative properties.
- **Omega-3 Fatty Acids**: Omega-3 fatty acid supplements, such as fish oil or flaxseed oil, have anti-inflammatory properties that may help reduce inflammation and support cardiovascular health in

individuals with diverticulosis.

Mind-Body Practices

Mind-body practices such as meditation, yoga, and acupuncture are integral components of integrative medicine approaches to diverticulosis management. These practices promote relaxation, stress reduction, and mind-body awareness, offering potential benefits for symptom relief and overall well-being.

- **Meditation**: Incorporate mindfulness meditation, guided imagery, or deep breathing exercises into daily routines to reduce stress, promote relaxation, and alleviate symptoms of diverticulosis.
- **Yoga**: Practice gentle yoga sequences, restorative poses, or yoga nidra (yogic sleep) to improve flexibility, reduce tension, and support gastrointestinal health in individuals with diverticulosis.
- **Acupuncture**: Consider acupuncture treatments from qualified practitioners to alleviate abdominal discomfort, promote pain relief, and support emotional well-being in individuals with diverticulosis.

Other Holistic Therapies

Other holistic therapies may complement conventional medical treatments and enhance overall well-being in individuals with diverticulosis. These therapies include:

- **Massage Therapy**: Massage therapy can help alleviate muscle tension, promote relaxation, and reduce stress levels in individuals with diverticulosis. Choose gentle abdominal massage techniques to support gastrointestinal function and alleviate discomfort.
- **Herbal Medicine**: Consult with qualified herbalists or naturopathic practitioners for personalized herbal

remedies and formulations that may support gastrointestinal health, reduce inflammation, and alleviate symptoms of diverticulosis.
- **Aromatherapy**: Aromatherapy involves the use of essential oils derived from plants to promote relaxation, reduce stress, and alleviate symptoms of diverticulosis. Diffuse calming essential oils such as lavender, chamomile, or peppermint, or dilute them in carrier oils for topical application.

Conclusion

In conclusion, integrative medicine approaches offer a holistic and personalized approach to diverticulosis management, combining conventional medical treatments with complementary and alternative therapies to optimize health and well-being. By addressing dietary factors, lifestyle habits, stress management, herbal remedies, supplements, mind-body practices, and other holistic therapies, integrative approaches aim to alleviate symptoms, promote gut health, and prevent diverticular complications. Individualized treatment plans should be developed in collaboration with healthcare providers to incorporate evidence-based interventions and tailor recommendations to individual needs and preferences. Integrative medicine approaches empower individuals with diverticulosis to take an active role in their health and well-being, fostering a holistic approach to disease management and promoting optimal outcomes.

CHAPTER 9: PATIENT EDUCATION AND COUNSELING

Understanding Diverticulosis

Diverticulosis is a common gastrointestinal condition characterized by the presence of small pouches or sacs, called diverticula, that protrude from the weakened areas of the colon wall. While diverticulosis itself typically does not cause symptoms or complications, understanding its underlying mechanisms, risk factors, and potential implications is essential for effective management and prevention. This section provides an in-depth exploration of diverticulosis, covering its definition, etiology, pathophysiology, risk factors, and clinical significance.

Definition

Diverticulosis refers to the presence of diverticula, small sac-like protrusions, along the inner lining of the colon, particularly in the sigmoid colon. These pouches develop when weak areas in the muscular wall of the colon balloon outward, forming small pockets that can vary in size and number. Diverticula are typically asymptomatic and are often discovered incidentally during diagnostic imaging or colonoscopy. Diverticulosis should be distinguished from diverticulitis, which occurs when diverticula become inflamed or infected, leading to symptoms and potential complications.

Etiology

The exact cause of diverticulosis is not fully understood, but several factors contribute to its development:

1. **Colonic Wall Weakness**: Diverticula form at sites of colonic wall weakness, where the inner layer of the colon protrudes through the outer muscular layer. Chronic pressure and strain on these weakened areas lead to the formation of diverticular pouches over time.
2. **Increased Intraluminal Pressure**: High intraluminal pressure within the colon, often due to constipation, inadequate fiber intake, or abnormal bowel habits, exacerbates colonic wall stress and contributes to diverticula formation.
3. **Dietary Factors**: Low-fiber diets, high intake of refined carbohydrates, and processed foods are associated with an increased risk of diverticulosis. Inadequate fiber intake leads to decreased stool bulk, prolonged transit time, and increased colonic pressure, predisposing to diverticular formation.
4. **Age**: Diverticulosis is more common with advancing age, particularly in individuals over 50 years old. Age-related changes in colonic structure and function, along with cumulative exposure to risk factors, contribute to the increased prevalence of diverticula among older adults.

Pathophysiology

The pathophysiology of diverticulosis involves complex

interactions between colonic wall structure, intraluminal pressure dynamics, gut microbiota, genetic factors, and environmental influences:

1. **Intestinal Wall Structure**: The colon consists of several layers, including the mucosa, submucosa, muscularis propria, and serosa. Diverticula form when weak areas in the muscular layer of the colon allow the mucosal layer to herniate outward, creating small pouches or sacs.
2. **Pressure Dynamics**: Increased intraluminal pressure within the colon, resulting from factors such as constipation, straining during bowel movements, and low-fiber diets, contributes to the formation and progression of diverticula. Chronic pressure and mechanical stress on weakened areas of the colon lead to the development of diverticular pouches over time.
3. **Microbiota Interaction**: Alterations in the gut microbiota composition and function may play a role in diverticulosis pathogenesis. Dysbiosis, or imbalance in the microbial community, can lead to inflammation, mucosal injury, and impaired colonic motility, predisposing to diverticular formation and progression.
4. **Genetic Factors**: Genetic predisposition may influence an individual's susceptibility to diverticulosis. Familial clustering and genetic polymorphisms associated with connective tissue disorders, such as Ehlers-Danlos syndrome and Marfan syndrome, have been implicated in diverticular disease.

Risk Factors

Several factors increase the risk of developing diverticulosis:

1. **Age**: The prevalence of diverticulosis increases with

age, particularly in individuals over 50 years old. Age-related changes in colonic structure and function, along with cumulative exposure to risk factors, contribute to the development of diverticular pouches.
2. **Dietary Factors**: Low-fiber diets, high intake of refined carbohydrates, and processed foods are associated with an increased risk of diverticulosis. Inadequate fiber intake leads to decreased stool bulk, prolonged transit time, and increased intraluminal pressure, predisposing to diverticular formation.
3. **Obesity**: Obesity and excess body weight are associated with an increased risk of diverticulosis. Abdominal adiposity and visceral fat accumulation contribute to elevated intra-abdominal pressure, impaired colonic motility, and greater mechanical stress on the colonic wall.
4. **Physical Inactivity**: Sedentary lifestyle and lack of regular physical activity are risk factors for diverticulosis. Reduced physical activity levels contribute to sluggish colonic motility, prolonged transit time, and increased intraluminal pressure, predisposing to diverticular formation.
5. **Smoking**: Smoking is a modifiable risk factor for diverticulosis. Cigarette smoking is associated with increased colonic wall tension, impaired microcirculation, and alterations in gut microbiota composition, contributing to the development and progression of diverticular disease.

Clinical Significance

While diverticulosis itself is typically asymptomatic and benign, it can have clinical significance due to its potential complications and associated conditions:

1. **Diverticulitis**: Diverticulitis occurs when diverticula

become inflamed or infected, leading to symptoms such as abdominal pain, fever, nausea, and changes in bowel habits. Complications of diverticulitis include abscess formation, perforation, fistula formation, and bowel obstruction, which may require medical intervention or surgical management.
2. **Bleeding**: Diverticulosis can predispose to diverticular bleeding, characterized by sudden onset of painless rectal bleeding, often associated with fresh red blood in the stool. Diverticular bleeding results from rupture of small blood vessels within diverticula and may require hospitalization and intervention to control bleeding.
3. **Symptomatic Diverticular Disease**: Some individuals with diverticulosis may experience symptomatic diverticular disease, characterized by recurrent abdominal pain, bloating, and changes in bowel habits. While the exact mechanisms underlying symptomatic diverticular disease are not fully understood, dietary factors, gut microbiota dysbiosis, and visceral hypersensitivity may play contributory roles.

Understanding the clinical significance of diverticulosis, along with its potential complications and associated conditions, is crucial for healthcare providers to effectively manage and counsel individuals with this condition. By addressing modifiable risk factors, promoting healthy lifestyle habits, and providing appropriate surveillance and management of complications, healthcare providers can optimize outcomes and quality of life for individuals with diverticulosis.

9.2 Lifestyle Modifications for Diverticulosis Management

Lifestyle modifications play a critical role in the management of diverticulosis, aiming to optimize gastrointestinal health, alleviate symptoms, and reduce the risk of diverticular complications. By adopting healthy lifestyle habits, individuals with diverticulosis can support bowel regularity, promote gut motility, and reduce intraluminal pressure within the colon. This section explores various lifestyle modifications that may benefit individuals with diverticulosis, including dietary changes, physical activity, stress management, and smoking cessation.

Dietary Modifications

1. **High-Fiber Diet**: Increase dietary fiber intake to promote bowel regularity and prevent constipation, a common risk factor for diverticulosis. Consume a variety of fiber-rich foods such as fruits, vegetables, whole grains, legumes, and nuts. Aim for at least 25-30 grams of fiber per day, gradually increasing fiber intake to avoid gastrointestinal discomfort.
2. **Fluid Intake**: Stay well-hydrated by drinking plenty of fluids, particularly water, to soften stool consistency and facilitate smooth bowel transit. Aim for adequate daily fluid intake, approximately 8-10 cups (2-2.5 liters) of water per day, or more as needed based on individual hydration needs and activity level.
3. **Healthy Fats**: Incorporate healthy fats such as omega-3 fatty acids found in fatty fish, flaxseeds, chia seeds, and walnuts. Omega-3 fatty acids have anti-inflammatory properties and may help reduce inflammation in the colon, supporting gastrointestinal health in individuals with diverticulosis.
4. **Limit Red Meat and Processed Foods**: Reduce consumption of red meat, processed meats, and high-

fat foods, which may contribute to inflammation and increase the risk of diverticular complications. Choose lean protein sources such as poultry, fish, legumes, and plant-based proteins more frequently.
5. **Probiotics and Prebiotics**: Include probiotic-rich foods (e.g., yogurt, kefir, fermented vegetables) and prebiotic-containing foods (e.g., garlic, onions, leeks, asparagus, bananas) in your diet to support a healthy gut microbiota. Probiotics help restore microbial balance, while prebiotics provide fuel for beneficial bacteria.

Physical Activity

1. **Regular Exercise**: Engage in regular physical activity to promote gastrointestinal motility, reduce constipation, and support overall health and well-being. Aim for at least 150 minutes of moderate-intensity aerobic exercise per week, such as brisk walking, cycling, swimming, or dancing.
2. **Abdominal Exercises**: Incorporate exercises that target the abdominal muscles, such as core strengthening exercises and yoga poses, to support abdominal tone and promote bowel function. Avoid excessive straining during abdominal exercises to prevent exacerbation of diverticular symptoms.

Stress Management

1. **Stress Reduction Techniques**: Practice stress reduction techniques such as meditation, deep breathing exercises, progressive muscle relaxation, or mindfulness practices to manage stress levels and promote relaxation. Stress management techniques help mitigate the effects of psychological stress on gastrointestinal function and overall well-being.

2. **Mind-Body Practices**: Explore mind-body practices such as yoga, tai chi, or qigong, which integrate physical movement with breath awareness and mindfulness. These practices promote relaxation, reduce muscle tension, and enhance mind-body awareness, fostering a sense of calm and balance.

Smoking Cessation

1. **Quit Smoking**: If you smoke, seek support and resources to quit smoking, as smoking is associated with an increased risk of diverticulosis and diverticular complications. Smoking cessation improves gastrointestinal health, reduces inflammation, and supports overall well-being.
2. **Nicotine Replacement Therapy**: Consider nicotine replacement therapy (e.g., nicotine patches, gum, lozenges) or prescription medications to help manage nicotine withdrawal symptoms and support smoking cessation efforts. Consult with healthcare providers or smoking cessation programs for personalized guidance and support.

Weight Management

1. **Maintain a Healthy Weight**: Achieve and maintain a healthy weight through a balanced diet, regular exercise, and lifestyle modifications. Excess body weight, particularly abdominal adiposity, is associated with an increased risk of diverticulosis and diverticular complications.
2. **Portion Control**: Practice portion control and mindful eating to prevent overeating and promote satiety. Choose nutrient-dense foods, incorporate plenty of fruits and vegetables, and limit high-calorie, low-nutrient foods to support weight management and

gastrointestinal health.

By implementing these lifestyle modifications, individuals with diverticulosis can optimize their gastrointestinal health, alleviate symptoms, and reduce the risk of diverticular complications. Consistency and adherence to these lifestyle changes are key to achieving long-term benefits and improving overall quality of life. Additionally, individuals should consult with healthcare providers or registered dietitians for personalized recommendations and guidance based on individual needs and preferences.

9.3 Monitoring and Follow-Up in Diverticulosis Management

Monitoring and follow-up care are essential components of diverticulosis management, aimed at assessing symptom progression, identifying complications, and adjusting treatment strategies as needed. Regular monitoring allows healthcare providers to track disease progression, evaluate treatment efficacy, and provide ongoing support to individuals with diverticulosis. This section outlines key aspects of monitoring and follow-up care for individuals with diverticulosis, including surveillance strategies, symptom assessment, and communication with healthcare providers.

Surveillance Strategies

1. **Colonoscopy**: Periodic colonoscopy may be recommended for individuals with diverticulosis, particularly if they are at higher risk of colorectal cancer or other gastrointestinal conditions. Colonoscopy allows healthcare providers to visualize the colon, assess diverticular changes, and screen for

polyps or other abnormalities.
2. **Imaging Studies**: In some cases, imaging studies such as computed tomography (CT) scans or magnetic resonance imaging (MRI) may be used to evaluate diverticular disease, assess complications, or monitor treatment response. These imaging modalities provide detailed anatomical information and help guide clinical decision-making.
3. **Symptom Monitoring**: Regular assessment of symptoms is crucial for monitoring disease progression and treatment response in individuals with diverticulosis. Healthcare providers should inquire about symptoms such as abdominal pain, changes in bowel habits, rectal bleeding, or other gastrointestinal complaints during follow-up visits.

Assessment of Complications

1. **Diverticulitis**: Individuals with diverticulosis should be monitored for signs and symptoms of diverticulitis, including abdominal pain, fever, nausea, vomiting, and changes in bowel habits. Prompt evaluation and management of diverticulitis episodes are essential to prevent complications such as abscess formation, perforation, or fistula formation.
2. **Diverticular Bleeding**: Monitoring for signs of diverticular bleeding, such as sudden onset of painless rectal bleeding or blood in the stool, is important for early detection and intervention. Diverticular bleeding can be severe and may require hospitalization, blood transfusion, or endoscopic hemostasis.
3. **Other Complications**: Healthcare providers should assess for other potential complications of diverticulosis, such as fistula formation, bowel obstruction, or colonic perforation. Prompt

recognition and management of these complications are essential to prevent serious morbidity and mortality.

Communication with Healthcare Providers

1. **Follow-Up Visits**: Schedule regular follow-up visits with healthcare providers to assess disease progression, review treatment efficacy, and address any concerns or questions. Follow-up intervals may vary based on individual risk factors, symptoms, and treatment response.
2. **Symptom Reporting**: Individuals with diverticulosis should promptly report any new or worsening symptoms to their healthcare providers. This includes abdominal pain, rectal bleeding, changes in bowel habits, fever, or other gastrointestinal symptoms that may indicate diverticular complications.
3. **Medication Management**: Healthcare providers should review medication regimens regularly, adjust dosages as needed, and monitor for potential side effects or drug interactions. Compliance with prescribed medications and lifestyle recommendations should be reinforced during follow-up visits.
4. **Dietary Counseling**: Registered dietitians or nutritionists can provide dietary counseling and support for individuals with diverticulosis. Regular dietary assessments and adjustments may be necessary to optimize fiber intake, manage symptoms, and promote gastrointestinal health.

Patient Education and Empowerment

1. **Self-Monitoring**: Encourage individuals with diverticulosis to engage in self-monitoring of

symptoms and overall well-being. Keeping a symptom diary or journal can help track symptom patterns, identify triggers, and monitor treatment response over time.

2. **Lifestyle Modifications**: Reinforce the importance of adherence to lifestyle modifications, including dietary changes, regular exercise, stress management, smoking cessation, and weight management. Empower individuals to take an active role in their health and well-being by adopting healthy lifestyle habits.

3. **Symptom Recognition**: Educate individuals about the signs and symptoms of diverticular complications, such as diverticulitis, diverticular bleeding, or other gastrointestinal emergencies. Provide guidance on when to seek medical attention and when to contact healthcare providers for evaluation and management.

4. **Follow-Up Care Planning**: Collaborate with individuals to develop personalized follow-up care plans based on their individual needs, preferences, and treatment goals. Emphasize the importance of regular monitoring, open communication, and shared decision-making in optimizing outcomes and quality of life.

By implementing a comprehensive approach to monitoring and follow-up care, healthcare providers can effectively manage diverticulosis, prevent complications, and support individuals in achieving optimal gastrointestinal health and well-being. Regular surveillance, symptom assessment, communication, and patient education are essential components of holistic diverticulosis management.

9.4 Addressing Psychological Impact of Diverticulosis

Diverticulosis, while often asymptomatic, can have a significant psychological impact on affected individuals. The chronic nature of the condition, potential for complications, and uncertainty about future health outcomes may lead to anxiety, stress, and concerns about quality of life. Addressing the psychological impact of diverticulosis is essential for comprehensive patient care and overall well-being. This section explores strategies for supporting individuals with diverticulosis from a psychological perspective, including education, counseling, coping techniques, and peer support.

Education and Information

1. **Patient Education**: Provide comprehensive education about diverticulosis, including its causes, symptoms, treatment options, and potential complications. Empower individuals with knowledge and understanding of their condition to alleviate fears and uncertainties.
2. **Clear Communication**: Foster open and honest communication with patients, addressing their concerns, answering questions, and providing reassurance about prognosis and management. Clarify misconceptions and dispel myths surrounding diverticulosis to reduce anxiety and uncertainty.

Counseling and Support

1. **Individual Counseling**: Offer individual counseling sessions with healthcare providers, psychologists, or

mental health professionals to address psychological distress related to diverticulosis. Provide a safe space for individuals to express their concerns, fears, and emotions about their health condition.
2. **Cognitive Behavioral Therapy (CBT)**: Utilize cognitive-behavioral techniques to help individuals identify and challenge negative thought patterns, manage stress, and develop coping strategies for dealing with the psychological impact of diverticulosis. CBT can empower individuals to adopt more adaptive ways of thinking and coping with their condition.
3. **Support Groups**: Connect individuals with diverticulosis to peer support groups or online communities where they can share experiences, exchange information, and receive encouragement from others facing similar challenges. Peer support can provide validation, understanding, and solidarity, reducing feelings of isolation and anxiety.

Coping Techniques

1. **Stress Management**: Teach stress reduction techniques such as deep breathing exercises, progressive muscle relaxation, mindfulness meditation, or guided imagery to help individuals manage anxiety and stress related to their health condition. Encourage regular practice of these techniques as part of a holistic self-care routine.
2. **Positive Coping Strategies**: Encourage the use of positive coping strategies such as problem-solving, seeking social support, engaging in enjoyable activities, and maintaining a sense of humor. Emphasize the importance of focusing on what individuals can control and taking proactive steps to manage their health and well-being.

Mind-Body Practices

1. **Mindfulness and Meditation**: Introduce mindfulness-based practices and meditation techniques to promote present-moment awareness, acceptance, and emotional resilience in individuals with diverticulosis. Mindfulness can help individuals cultivate a sense of calm, reduce rumination, and enhance psychological well-being.
2. **Yoga and Relaxation Exercises**: Recommend gentle yoga practices, relaxation exercises, or gentle stretching routines to promote relaxation, relieve tension, and improve mind-body awareness. Yoga can be particularly beneficial for reducing stress, enhancing flexibility, and fostering a sense of inner peace.

Promoting Self-Efficacy and Empowerment

1. **Goal Setting**: Collaborate with individuals to set realistic goals for managing their diverticulosis and improving overall well-being. Encourage small, achievable steps toward positive health behaviors and self-care practices.
2. **Self-Monitoring**: Encourage individuals to track their symptoms, emotions, and coping strategies using a journal or diary. Self-monitoring can help individuals identify triggers, patterns, and progress over time, empowering them to take an active role in their health management.

Holistic Supportive Care

1. **Integrated Care Approach**: Adopt an integrated care approach that addresses the physical, psychological, and social aspects of diverticulosis management.

Collaborate with interdisciplinary healthcare team members, including gastroenterologists, primary care providers, psychologists, dietitians, and social workers, to provide holistic supportive care.

2. **Patient-Centered Care**: Tailor interventions and support services to meet the individual needs, preferences, and cultural backgrounds of individuals with diverticulosis. Recognize the unique challenges and strengths of each patient and provide personalized care that promotes autonomy, dignity, and self-empowerment.

By addressing the psychological impact of diverticulosis and providing comprehensive support, healthcare providers can enhance the overall well-being and quality of life of individuals living with this condition. Empowering patients with knowledge, counseling support, coping techniques, and holistic care fosters resilience, adaptation, and psychological thriving in the face of chronic health challenges.

CHAPTER 10: FUTURE DIRECTIONS IN DIVERTICULOSIS RESEARCH

10.1 Emerging Therapies for Diverticulosis

As our understanding of diverticulosis continues to evolve, researchers and clinicians are exploring novel therapeutic approaches aimed at improving symptom management, preventing complications, and enhancing overall gastrointestinal health. Emerging therapies for diverticulosis encompass a range of interventions, including pharmacological agents, dietary supplements, minimally invasive procedures, and innovative technologies. This section provides an overview of promising emerging therapies that hold potential for the management of diverticulosis.

1. Mesalamine and Anti-Inflammatory Agents

Mesalamine, a 5-aminosalicylic acid derivative commonly used in the treatment of inflammatory bowel diseases (IBD), has shown promise in the management of symptomatic uncomplicated diverticular disease (SUDD). Studies have demonstrated that mesalamine may help reduce inflammation, modulate immune responses, and improve symptoms such as abdominal pain and bloating in individuals with SUDD. Other anti-inflammatory agents, such as corticosteroids and tumor necrosis factor-alpha (TNF-α) inhibitors, are also being investigated for their potential role in diverticulosis management, particularly in cases of diverticulitis.

2. Probiotics and Prebiotics

Probiotics and prebiotics have emerged as promising adjunctive therapies for diverticulosis management, aiming to restore microbial balance, promote gut health, and reduce the risk of diverticular complications. Probiotic supplements containing beneficial bacteria such as Lactobacillus and Bifidobacterium strains have been shown to modulate gut microbiota composition, enhance immune function, and reduce inflammation in animal and human studies. Prebiotics, non-digestible fibers that serve as fuel for beneficial bacteria, may also exert beneficial effects on gut microbiota composition and function.

3. Fiber Supplements and Bulking Agents

Fiber supplements and bulking agents play a crucial role in the management of diverticulosis by promoting bowel regularity, softening stool consistency, and reducing intraluminal pressure within the colon. Emerging formulations of fiber supplements, such as psyllium husk, methylcellulose, and wheat dextrin, offer convenient and effective options for individuals with diverticulosis who may have difficulty achieving adequate dietary fiber intake. These supplements help optimize gastrointestinal motility, prevent constipation, and minimize diverticular symptoms.

4. Endoscopic Therapies

Endoscopic therapies have emerged as minimally invasive approaches for the management of diverticular disease, offering potential benefits such as symptom relief, complication prevention, and mucosal healing. Endoscopic interventions such as endoscopic band ligation, endoscopic clipping, and endoscopic suturing aim to seal off diverticular necks, reduce luminal pressure, and prevent diverticular bleeding or recurrent episodes of diverticulitis. These techniques may be particularly beneficial for individuals with recurrent diverticular complications or persistent symptoms despite conservative management.

5. Fecal Microbiota Transplantation (FMT)

Fecal microbiota transplantation (FMT) represents a novel therapeutic approach for diverticulosis management, leveraging the potential of gut microbiota modulation to restore microbial balance, reduce inflammation, and improve gastrointestinal health. FMT involves the transfer of fecal material from healthy donors to individuals with gastrointestinal disorders, including diverticular disease, with the goal of replenishing beneficial bacteria and restoring microbial diversity. Preliminary studies have shown promising results in terms of symptom improvement and reduction of diverticular complications following FMT interventions.

6. Novel Imaging Modalities

Advancements in imaging technologies offer new opportunities for the early detection, characterization, and monitoring of diverticular disease. Emerging imaging modalities such as magnetic resonance imaging (MRI), contrast-enhanced ultrasound (CEUS), and virtual colonoscopy (CT colonography) provide detailed anatomical information, functional assessment, and visualization of diverticular changes in the colon. These non-invasive imaging techniques offer potential advantages such as improved patient comfort, reduced radiation exposure, and enhanced diagnostic accuracy compared to traditional imaging modalities.

7. Biofeedback Therapy

Biofeedback therapy has emerged as a non-pharmacological approach for the management of diverticular symptoms, particularly in cases of pelvic floor dysfunction and dyssynergic defecation. Biofeedback techniques involve real-time monitoring and feedback of pelvic floor muscle activity, bowel motility, and defecation dynamics to promote optimal coordination and relaxation of pelvic floor muscles during defecation. Biofeedback therapy aims to improve rectal sensation, coordination, and evacuation dynamics, leading to enhanced bowel function and symptom relief in individuals with diverticulosis.

8. Novel Drug Targets

Research efforts are underway to identify novel drug targets and therapeutic agents that target key pathophysiological mechanisms underlying diverticulosis. Potential targets include mucosal inflammation, colonic wall integrity, gut microbiota dysbiosis, and visceral hypersensitivity. Novel pharmacological agents such as selective cytokine inhibitors, anti-fibrotic agents, gut microbiota modulators, and neuromodulators hold promise for the future development of targeted therapies for diverticular disease.

Conclusion

Emerging therapies for diverticulosis represent a dynamic and evolving field of research and innovation, offering new opportunities for the management of this common gastrointestinal condition. From pharmacological agents and dietary supplements to minimally invasive procedures and innovative technologies, these emerging therapies hold promise for improving symptom management, preventing complications, and enhancing overall gastrointestinal health in individuals with diverticulosis. Continued research, clinical trials, and collaboration among researchers, clinicians, and industry stakeholders are essential to advance the field and translate promising therapies into clinical practice.

10.2 Precision Medicine in Diverticulosis Management

Precision medicine, also known as personalized medicine, is a paradigm shift in healthcare that aims to tailor medical treatment and interventions to individual patients based on their unique genetic, environmental, and lifestyle factors. In the context of diverticulosis management, precision medicine holds great promise for optimizing patient outcomes, enhancing treatment efficacy, and reducing the risk of complications. This section explores the principles of precision medicine and its potential applications in the management of diverticulosis.

1. Genetic Profiling

Genetic profiling enables the identification of genetic variants and polymorphisms associated with diverticulosis susceptibility, disease progression, and treatment response. Advances in genomic sequencing technologies allow for the comprehensive analysis of an individual's genetic makeup, including single nucleotide polymorphisms (SNPs), copy number variations (CNVs), and gene expression profiles. By elucidating the genetic basis of diverticular disease, clinicians can stratify patients based on their genetic risk profiles and tailor treatment strategies accordingly.

2. Biomarker Discovery

Biomarker discovery efforts aim to identify novel molecular markers and biological indicators associated with diverticulosis pathogenesis, disease activity, and prognosis. Biomarkers may include circulating proteins, metabolites, inflammatory markers, microbial signatures, and genetic markers that reflect underlying disease processes and treatment response. By monitoring biomarker profiles, clinicians can assess disease progression, predict treatment outcomes, and guide therapeutic decision-making in individuals with diverticulosis.

3. Microbiome Analysis

The gut microbiome plays a crucial role in diverticulosis pathogenesis and disease progression, influencing colonic inflammation, mucosal integrity, and immune function. Precision medicine approaches leverage microbiome analysis techniques such as metagenomic sequencing, 16S rRNA profiling, and metabolomic analysis to characterize microbial communities and functional pathways associated with diverticular disease. By assessing individual microbiome profiles, clinicians can identify microbial signatures, dysbiosis patterns, and microbial biomarkers that inform targeted interventions, such as probiotic supplementation, dietary modification, or microbiota-targeted therapies.

4. Dietary and Nutritional Optimization

Precision nutrition approaches tailor dietary recommendations and nutritional interventions to individual patient characteristics, including genetic predisposition, gut microbiome composition, metabolic status, and dietary preferences. By integrating genetic, microbial, and metabolic data, clinicians can design personalized dietary plans that optimize nutrient intake, modulate gut microbiota composition, and mitigate dietary risk factors associated with diverticulosis development and progression. Precision nutrition strategies may include personalized fiber prescriptions, microbiota-targeted diets, and supplementation with specific nutrients or dietary components.

5. Pharmacogenomics

Pharmacogenomics involves the study of how genetic variations influence drug metabolism, efficacy, and adverse drug reactions. In the context of diverticulosis management, pharmacogenomic approaches enable the selection of pharmacological agents and dosages based on individual genetic profiles, optimizing treatment response and minimizing adverse effects. By considering genetic factors such as drug metabolism enzymes, drug transporters, and drug targets, clinicians can personalize pharmacotherapy regimens for individuals with diverticular disease, maximizing therapeutic benefits and minimizing risks.

6. Digital Health Technologies

Digital health technologies, including mobile health apps, wearable devices, and telehealth platforms, facilitate remote monitoring, real-time data collection, and patient engagement in diverticulosis management. These digital tools enable individuals to track symptoms, monitor dietary intake, record medication adherence, and communicate with healthcare providers from the convenience of their homes. By leveraging digital health technologies, clinicians can gather longitudinal data, identify disease trends, and provide timely interventions tailored to individual patient needs, enhancing the efficiency and effectiveness of diverticulosis care delivery.

Conclusion

Precision medicine holds tremendous potential for revolutionizing the management of diverticulosis by shifting from a one-size-fits-all approach to personalized, patient-centered care. By integrating genomic, microbial, dietary, and clinical data, clinicians can tailor treatment strategies, dietary recommendations, and lifestyle interventions to individual patient characteristics, optimizing outcomes and quality of life for individuals with diverticular disease. Continued research, collaboration, and innovation in the field of precision medicine are essential for translating these promising approaches into clinical practice and improving patient care in diverticulosis management.

Made in United States
Troutdale, OR
09/30/2024